Living Logotherapy

Published by

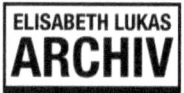

www.elisabeth-lukas-archiv.de

© 2021 Elisabeth-Lukas-Archiv gGmbH
Dr. Heidi Schönfeld
Nürnberger Straße 103a
D-96050 Bamberg
info@elisabeth-lukas-archiv.de

This English edition published in German as *Psychotherapie in Würde, Logotherapie konkret* © 2020 Elisabeth-Lukas-Archiv gGmbH, Bamberg

Elisabeth Lukas, Heidi Schönfeld
Psychotherapy with Dignity, Logotherapy in Action

Translated from the German by:
Dr. David Nolland, Oxford, and Dr. Heidi Schönfeld, Bamberg

Cover design, typesetting and layout:
Bernhard Keller, Köln

Print and distribution: tredition, Hamburg
ISBN **978-3-00-066694-0** (paperback)
ISBN **978-3-00-066693-3** (eBook)

Elisabeth Lukas – Heidi Schönfeld

PSYCHOTHERAPY WITH DIGNITY

Elisabeth Lukas – Heidi Schönfeld

Psychotherapy with Dignity
Logotherapy in Action

LIVING LOGOTHERAPY

A publication series of the Elisabeth-Lukas-Archive

Contents

Foreword for the Series "Living Logotherapy"

"In our time, people usually have enough to live on. What they often lack, however, is something to live for." This is how Viktor E. Frankl, the Viennese psychiatrist and founder of logotherapy, summarised a problem that is just as relevant today as ever. Elisabeth Lukas, a clinical psychologist and psychotherapist, has an international reputation as Frankl's most important student. In her many books, she illustrates how logotherapy provides help in cases of mental illness, enriches the everyday life of healthy people and inspires us all to lead a meaningful, fulfilling life. Her books illustrate how humane, authentic and up-to-date a "living logotherapy" can be. The main objective of this new series is to make her books, which have enjoyed lasting success in the German-speaking world, more accessible to speakers of English.

Many people have worked hard to make it possible for the Elisabeth Lukas Archive to publish this new series. Particular thanks are due to our translator Dr. David Nolland, who has produced a fluid text that remains very close to the original. He has excellent knowledge in the field of logotherapy and supervises this series in all matters relating to the English-speaking market. Thanks are also due to Prof. Dr. Alexander Batthyány, who supported us from the beginning and will accompany this series as a guide. The formatting and layout is due to Bernhard Keller, and the beautiful presentation of the books is wholly attributable to his expertise.

The first book in this series is a collaborative project combining discussions of the theory of logotherapy by Lukas with numerous case studies by Schönfeld, and the second book is a textbook by Elisabeth Lukas on the fundamental concepts of logotherapy and their applications.

This third book is a further collaboration between Lukas and Schönfeld. It mainly consists of case studies supplemented with theoretical analyses of how these cases illustrate the practical application of logotherapy. The book includes a short introduction to logotherapy and ends with discussions of a number of topics from a logotherapeutic perspective.

We sincerely hope that this practical guide to the application of logotherapeutic methods will be helpful and illuminating for English speaking practitioners and other interested parties and will clearly illustrate the effectiveness and applicability of logotherapy.

Dr. Heidi Schönfeld
Director of the Elisabeth-Lukas-Archive

Translator's Note

Logotherapy presents a particular challenge for the translator. Viktor Frankl's own works are full of humour and metaphor, and his distinctive way of making his point often relies heavily on wordplay, poetic forms of expression and nuances of language that combine colloquial language with philosophically suggestive formulations distilled from a profound understanding of the history of European thought. He coined a number of original terms and concepts that play a key role in his work. Frankl was often dissatisfied with the published translations of many of these key terms, and his own translations, where available, provide valuable clues to his thinking.

Elisabeth Lukas has a distinctive written style that shares the aforementioned features of Frankl's writing. She has continued in Frankl's footsteps linguistically as much as she has intellectually and spiritually. Frankl never saw the logotherapy he had originated as something finished and set in stone, but as a system of thought that should continually be developed in response to the inexhaustible insights into human nature arising from his focus on meaning and the possibilities of the human spirit. In this book, Elisabeth Lukas and Heidi Schönfeld have produced a remarkable testimony to how therapeutically effective this system of thought is in practice.

Translations of Frankl's works have, where possible, been taken from the standard editions of his works in English cited in the footnotes. Where this is not possible, I have cited the German editions, and the translations are my own.

I would also like to thank Heidi Schönfeld for her close collaboration in producing this translation. Without her help, an accurate and faithful English-language account of Frankl's methods in action would have been impossible.

Dr. David Nolland

A Brief Introduction
to Logotherapy

(Elisabeth Lukas interviewed by Bernd Ahrendt)

Bernd Ahrendt is a Professor of Business Administration, with a particular interest in human resources management, working at the FOM University in Hannover. In 2018, he travelled to Vienna to interview Elisabeth Lukas. Bernd Ahrendt has agreed for passages from his interview to be reprinted here to provide readers with an introduction to the basic concepts of logotherapy.

Ahrendt: Prof. Lukas, could you sum up the essence of logotherapy in a few words?

Lukas: Viktor Emil Frankl, born in 1905, began his research as a young doctor with two basic questions that interested him as a prospective psychiatrist. The first question was: "What makes a human human? Is there anything that is unique to being human?" The second was: "What keeps humans psychically healthy, or enables them to get healthy again if they are ill?" The second question was particularly innovative in Frankl's time, because all the psychiatric experts of that time considered only the causes of becoming ill, and not the basis for getting healthy again.

To answer his first question, Frankl began to investigate the human "spirit", which, according to his definition, is the third dimension of being human. One should bear in mind that according to the philosophy current at that time, one only talked about the "body" (the first dimension) and the "soul" (the second dimension), and that in the developing field of psychology, the traditional concept of "soul" was simply translated as "psyche". So all of our cognitions and emotions were subsumed under the heading of psyche. This left out everything that is specifically human, because thoughts and feelings also exist to a certain extent for animals. If one wants to pick out what is uniquely human, one must venture into the third dimension, in which Frankl located phenomena such as our (potential) freedom of will and responsibility, our ethical and artistic sensibilities, and our search for meaning and our yearning for an ultimate meaning (God?). These phenomena take us beyond the horizon of the animal world, and in a modern context also beyond the horizon of intelligent computers and robots.

To answer his second question Frankl discovered the immense significance of one's perspective on meaning for the stability of the human psyche (and body). It is precisely when life becomes difficult that it becomes decisively important whether one sees a meaning in continuing to live. But even in comfortable circumstances, life becomes less satisfying when it is empty of meaning. In the light of these two groundbreaking realisations, Frankl founded his "meaning-centred psychotherapy", which he called "logotherapy". It can be seen as a "psychotherapy from the spiritual and towards the spiritual".

Ahrendt: What did Frankl find in the course of his research?

Lukas: In the 1930s, Frankl worked at the psychiatric hospital "Am Steinhof" in Vienna. There he had the opportunity to talk with hundreds of sick and severely depressive people. Amongst other things, he heard about the hardships of their childhoods, about their disappointments and psychic injuries. It was there that he had the idea to carry out a controlled experiment, in which he interviewed numerous healthy people (doctors, nurses, students) and found that these inconspicuous and psychically "normal" people, who were pursuing their professions and getting on with their daily lives without difficulty, had typically had just as many traumas, disappointments and injuries in their lives as his patients. As a result, Frankl abandoned Sigmund

Freud's trauma theory. He recognised that there are certainly patho-genic, that is, illness-causing factors in life, but at the same time there are also protective factors. And that when enough protective factors are present, the illness-causing factors become less danger-ous. This thesis is now undisputed. It has been known for a long time from general medicine that, for example, infections have an effect when a person's immune system is already weak, and cause little damage when the organism's resistance to illness is well-developed. In the psychic domain, a person's inner meaning fulfilment is one of the most powerful protective factors. Frankl deduced from this that any form of finding and fulfilling meaning contributes to psychic healing. It can be seen from his many well-documented case studies that this really works in practice.

I would like to add one more thing: recent resilience studies have confirmed Frankl's discoveries 100%. People who pick themselves up after a severe blow of fate has knocked them down, do so on the basis of affirming a particular meaning perspective. Instead of al-ways looking back on what they have suffered, they live primarily in the present, which they shape as best they can according to a value-oriented vision of the future. In this way they rescue themselves from the unhealthy miasma of their trauma (much as Baron Münchhausen pulled himself out of a swamp by his own ponytail).

Ahrendt: But then why are so many people stuck in their negatively perceived past?

Lukas: There are many explanations for this. It is easier to complain about something than to make it better, it is easier to blame someone else than to do something on one's own initiative, and so on. The way of thinking of traditional psychoanalysis is also partly responsible for our unhelpful tendency to look backwards. It has propagated the idea of delving into the past. But I do not want to blame psychotherapy, because it is a very new discipline, only about 120 years old. Every evolutionary process proceeds by trial and error, and this has also been the case with psychotherapy. Therapeutic methods have been developed one after another, always needing to be corrected. Frankl himself was an important corrector. Meanwhile, the psychoanalytic illusion that a psychic illness will disappear when its causes are discovered has melted away. Strategies based on uncovering causes have not proved successful, quite apart from the part that they are usually associated with too much unprovable speculation.

Ahrendt: Does this also have to do with the fact that there is often more than one cause that leads or can lead to a psychic illness?

Lukas: The progress made in neurobiology and psychology since Freud's time has shown that the causes of illness are closely interrelated. Genetic research has revealed that many more psychic conditions than we thought can be traced back to genetic predispositions. One does not only inherit blonde hair or blue eyes from one's genes, one also inherits character dispositions such as a tendency to addiction, hysteria or depression. This does not mean that the corresponding illness will necessarily occur, only that one should be careful in certain situations. These endogenous dispositions interact with exogenous influences, and not just from parents and teachers. The media also has a powerful influence, and the effect of societal trends should not be underestimated.

But all this is still not the heart of the matter. For amongst all these diverse influences is the human capacity for self-determination, which shapes each person as an individual. Even children already have their own personalities and make their own individual choices. Although the spiritual dimension in little people is still partly dormant or not yet fully developed, it still permeates the psychophysical level and helps to determine what the little person becomes. Children are not determined by how they are brought up by their parents, and adults are not pure victims of their past circumstances.

Ahrendt: This would mean that all people have a significant influence on their own lives. Even as a child, but also as an adult.

Lukas: Yes. According to a famous analogy by Frankl, a person is like a builder. Genetic predispositions and the various influences from one's environment form the building material that each person has to work with. Unfortunately this building material is not fairly distributed. Some inhabitants of this world have excellent building material: loving parents, a healthy body, they live in a peaceful country. Others have inferior building materials available: an antisocial milieu, poverty or the ravages of war. This is when the third dimension comes into play: the builder uses this material in a unique way. And one finds that some builders who have been given the best marble blocks to work with (an outstanding musical talent or a superb role model for loving behaviour, for example) leave these blocks unworked and squander their time away. Other builders, who have been assigned only crumbly sandstone (for example a low birth weight or poor educational opportunities) use them to build a cosy cottage or a pretty chapel by the wayside. Frankl said, "Man is the being who always decides." And what does he decide? "What he will be in the next moment."

Ahrendt: You have told us about the concept of meaning, which plays a big role in Frankl's terminology. Could you explain this term in more detail?

Lukas: First, I would like to differentiate between the concept of "meaning" and the concept of "values". Values are "meaning universals". Meaning, on the other hand, is unique. This means that the "meaning of the moment", as Frankl calls it, always exists with reference to a particular person in a particular set of circumstances. It is the optimal result (for all people involved) that *this particular person* can achieve in *this particular situation*. What one is "called" to, so to

17

speak. To illustrate this with the two of us: for me the "meaning of the moment" is to answer your questions as well as I can. If I, for example, said, "The weather is beautiful today, Professor, so I think it would be meaningful to take a walk," you would answer, "No, Mrs Lukas, that would not be meaningful at this time. I have travelled all the way from Germany to interview you. You agreed to this. So what is meaningful is to sit here and continue to talk with me!" What this example shows is that although a pleasant walk on a sunny day certainly has a value, this value is not what is important right now. It is not its turn to be actualised. Later this afternoon, after we have said goodbye, it may be very meaningful to go for a walk before bed instead of continuing to sit here.

Likewise, the "meaning of the moment" is different for each person. Later, when you leave me, something different will be waiting for you than for me. In other words, *meaning is ever-present, and ever-different.* As long as we are conscious, there exists some meaningful possibility for us, whatever our situation. People who have a well-developed system of values, who acknowledge many sources of value in their lives, naturally find it easier to discover the "meaning of the moment" than those for whom a single value is always in play. Nevertheless, they must take care to keep their other values waiting in their order of precedence and not be pressurised by them. And it is also important to remember that rest and leisure time also has a high value.

Ahrendt: What about the three categories of value that Frankl developed?

Lukas: Frankl spoke of three "main avenues of meaning-discovery": *creative values*, *experiential values* and *attitudinal values*. Creative values and experiential values are shared by almost everyone. They build a bridge between a person and the world. Creativity allows one to bring something new into the world. For example, a woman knits a sweater. She gives it to "the world" and she is happy if it fits the recipient well. In contrast, experiential values have to do with receiving something good from the world – the world gives something to us. This presupposes that we are open to receive this gift and that we know how to appreciate its value. For example, walking outdoors is only a valuable experience for someone who is receptive to the beauty of nature. People who stomp around complaining and pay no attention to the surrounding flowers and fields destroy the experiential value for themselves.

Then we have the attitudinal values. For Frankl, these were the highest possible values that can be actualised by a person, because they are the hardest to actualise. They have nothing to do with joy (as creative or experiential values do) but with suffering, because they can be chosen in the case of misfortune, loss of hope, or when people come up against insurmountable obstacles. If action can still be taken in such cases to improve the unfortunate situation, of course this action (inspired by creative values) takes precedence, it has the higher *priority*. If, for example, someone has lost his or her job, it is certainly meaningful to look for a new one. If, however, nothing more can be done to eliminate the misfortune, if one is confronted with unalterable suffering, for example on the loss of a loved one, then the question is how one bears and endures this suffering. One can always adopt various attitudes. One can wildly shout out one's anger and non-acceptance of fate, one can sink into dull despair, but one can also win through to an heroic acceptance of fate and in this way adopt a valuable attitude (actualise an attitudinal value). This value is *superior*. For example, someone may think, "I have received many good things in life. I enjoyed the company of the person I loved for many years, and I will be thankful for this, even if I am now alone. My love does not end with death, it remains alive in my heart…" This is a wonderful attitude to adopt in the face of mourning and loss.

The significance of attitudinal values is particularly apparent in the following context. According to the laws of biology, frustration automatically produces aggression. At the psychophysical-animalistic level, aggression is nothing more than a spurt of energy. If, for example, an animal is being hunted by another animal, this is a frustration in biological terminology, and the animal responds by becoming aggressive, that is, hormones are released which give it the energy to fight for survival or to flee. With humans, frustrations are usually psychic pressures that similarly give rise to aggression, but unlike animals, humans can choose what to do with the biological spurt of energy. Humans can also fight or flee, or even harm them-selves (which animals do not do), or they can transform their energy into an admirable attitude – in cases where it would not be meaning-ful to fight or to flee.

Ahrendt: But one does feel this enormous anger in oneself.

Lukas: Yes, that is true. This is why many people are tempted to let their anger out somehow, to direct it against someone. They are like a tiger in the zoo that attacks its keeper because it has a toothache. The toothache is not the keeper's fault! In technical language we call this a "displacement" (of the aggression onto the wrong person). But a human is *more* than a tiger, which is why displacements like this are unethical in human society. If a man who is annoyed at his boss comes home in the evening, kicks the dog and shouts at his wife, in other words if he takes out his feelings on the innocent and the unin-volved, it doesn't help him that much. He just adds to the suffering in the world, and it does not solve his problem. It is much better either to address the conflict constructively with his boss (actualising crea-tive values) for example by speaking out clearly, changing work priorities, etc. or – if there is no alternative – to adopt a positive atti-tude to the situation, for example by saying to himself that at least he has a job, that it is good that he can feed his family and he will learn how to handle the idiosyncrasies of his boss without losing his calm. This would be an admirable attitude for him to develop.

Ahrendt: You are asking a lot from people: on the one hand self-reflection, to allow one to recognise what is going on in the situation, and on the other endurance of suffering.

Lukas: I am not the one who is asking it; the *logos* is asking it. It is the only meaningful way to deal with pain and sorrow; everything else increases pain and sorrow, and this is the last thing we need as a human family.

I would like to add one more thing. True heroes are not people whose statues are on monuments, because they conquered lands and won battles, true heroes are often simple people. They are more common than you imagine, Professor Ahrendt. Countless people have the sensitivity to break the chain of suffering when necessary; one must recognise them and honour their achievements. Suppose a woman is lying in the hospital and can't sleep at night because of the pain of her wounds. In the morning a nurse comes into the room and the woman smiles and wishes her a good morning. What has happened there? The sick woman has undergone a terrible night, but she manages a friendly greeting. She has experienced something bad and yet she spreads goodness. *That* is heroism! And that – not just the perpetuation of evil – is within the capabilities of every person. It is not impossible to respond to a bad experience by spreading love – and this is what we are called to do by the *logos*.

Ahrendt: Do you mean that there is a higher power calling on us to do this? Calling us to work for good in the world?

Lukas: It does not matter what you call this mysterious "higher power". The fact is that humans are not the creators of everything. We are not the creators of meaning. We can only seek meaning with humility, find it, follow it or dismiss it, but we cannot twist its message around according to our own wishes. Frankl laconically remarked that it is not a case of what *we* can expect from life, but of what *life* expects from us. For the most part, we sense what is expected from us. If we are walking in the street and an elderly man falls on the pavement, we feel deep down what life expects from us in that moment. Of course we can just walk past the man who has fallen. Meaning cannot compel us to do anything. But it is clearly asking us to stop and help the fallen man.

Ahrendt: Are these not just moral ideas that I have picked up?

Lukas: They are, but this is not the whole story. As you grew up, you received guidance not just from those around you, but also from your human nature. You have a "meaning organ" – your conscience. There are many studies showing that people can calmly throw overboard the wisdom they were taught in childhood. People who were raised with strict moral views tend to rebel against them and revel in forbidden amusements. Others bravely walk away from a criminal household environment. As already discussed, it is the builder – the spiritual person – who oversees the work, whatever building material is at hand.

To be human means to have an agency in oneself that perceives the call of the logos. To be human also means to possess the power to decide whether to ignore this call or to make it one's guiding principle.

Ahrendt: But where does one learn how to do this? Where can I learn how to feel this power and to know what I am called to in a particular situation? What is the meaningful thing that I should be doing *now*, that is sometimes not centred on *me*, but on others?

Lukas: You are right that, from the point of view of meaning, the self is not the centre point of spiritual endeavours. The divide between selfishness and altruism, however, is an illusory one. If one wants to commit oneself to another person, one has to keep oneself in good shape. People who overwork massively and treat themselves like slaves are not behaving meaningfully – even if they are slaving away for the service of others. Their service will continually diminish in quality, as will their own competence. We are also familiar with the opposite evil: people who are only interested in themselves and their own welfare are sucked into an existential vacuum that robs them of joy in life. Soon they are bored by everything, because they are no longer good for anything or for anyone. Meaning is just the guardian of the balance between being for something or for someone, and carefully polishing up one's own being, to make it shine. Meaning is always meaning for everyone who is involved in a given life situation.

Ahrendt: Clearly this means that one must be sensitive enough to recognise the meaning in a situation, but it could also make it necessary to say no to someone else's wishes and thereby appear harsh to others.

Lukas: Have Faith, Professor! We humans are equipped with a profound sensitivity for meaning and values. Our biggest problem is not to perceive what is right, but to do it.

Ahrendt: But where does one get this trust? And what happens with someone whose parents have not provided them with basic trust?

Lukas: Stop! Who says that it is the parents who provide children with basic trust? Of course it is important and of lasting relevance whether parents provide their children with a safe nest. There is no doubt that adults who have experienced that safety at home find it easier to develop trust in others than those who have had to do without parental love and affection. But basic trust is a uniquely human phenomenon, which is an inalienable part of being human. It can be shaken by bad experiences, but it can never be completely extinguished. There is always a spark remaining, and through this basic trust can always be restored, whether with therapeutic help or through one's own efforts.

Ahrendt: But when I meet people who tell me that they have no basic trust...

Lukas: Then they are mistaken. Or they are just making excuses. For example, in court, people like to argue that criminal offences can be traced back to childhood neglect. One can accept this as a mitigating circumstance, but only with reservations. No person is a pre-programmed machine. Freedom and basic trust, conscience and individual responsibility are inalienable possessions, which are "breathed in with the Spirit," to express it biblically. This makes it possible for us not to capitulate in the face of unfavourable starting conditions. Statistics support this thesis more than they contradict it. Yes, there are many human disasters involving people who have had difficult histories. But also, a surprising percentage of neglected, abused, even exploited people have turned things around with the help of the "defiant power of the spirit" and have developed into decent, upright human beings.

Going back to basic trust, it is weakened today much more by noise and distractions than by bad childhood experiences. This generation is constantly exposed to audio-visual stimuli, and has hardly any opportunity for reflection. If one is uninterruptedly distracted by multitasking and staring at electronic screens, one cannot hear the quiet voice of one's inner feel for meaning. In order not to lose contact with this feel for meaning, one should regularly withdraw into silence, even if it is only for 10 to 15 minutes a day, in a place where one will not be disturbed. This is immensely fruitful.

Ahrendt: Does this make it possible to get one's basic trust back?

Lukas: At the very least, it leads to deeper insights. Basic trust does not suggest that everything will always go well. What it says is that everything has a hidden meaning, whether we understand it or not, whatever the outcome. It says that there exists an ultimate harmony that we cannot and do not need to grasp, that takes into account all our troubles and suffering, even guilt and death. Human beings need to believe in something, whether they want to or not. Even convinced atheists believe that there are deeper connections that are beyond human imagining, that transcend the boundaries of human knowledge. Anyone who recognises a boundary also recognises that there is something on the other side of the boundary, otherwise it would not be a boundary. Directly or indirectly, we all bow down before what is on this other side, even if we have no words or images for it.

Ahrendt: How can one win back basic trust?

Lukas: That is an interesting question, because we know analogous processes in psychotherapeutic practice. To achieve a desired goal, a sustained investment must be made. We have already seen this in our explanation of experiential values: one has to be innerly open to a value before one is able to live it out as a value. Anxiety disorders are a striking example of this. First, while one is still shaking with fear, one has to submit oneself to the imagined object of fear (for example in the case of a fear of flying one has to get into an airplane) in order to be able to live a life ultimately less constrained by fear. The same thing applies to addictions. First, while one is still addicted, one has to behave as if one were already free from addiction (one has to practise abstinence) in order to be ultimately free from addiction. Even in the case of interpersonal conflicts, "advance investments" of this sort, as they are called in logotherapy, are the only way to achieve peace. One first has to reach out a hand to one's enemy in order to be able to make the enemy into a friend. I have described this very briefly, but the principle is clear: without advance investments of courage, perseverance, humour, forbearance, one can expect no gain. The same principle applies to the winning back of basic trust: every advance investment of trust in life will be rewarded.

Ahrendt: You say that humour as well as courage is needed?

Lukas: Let us consider anxiety disorders again. Suppose that a man has an extreme fear of dogs, cynophobia. If he sees a dog in the distance, he either turns around or takes a detour. This is an indication that there is an advance investment to be made, which he can make easier with the use of humour. One should walk with him past a little dachshund (perhaps for the first time) to which he should (paradoxically) say, jokingly: "Go ahead, show your teeth! You won't get succulent legs like mine every day, so go ahead and enjoy them…!" The dachshund will probably run past without paying any attention. The man should whisper after it: "What a coward you are! You didn't even manage a small bite…" In this humorous way the man will gain the confidence to walk more and more often past bigger and bigger dogs.

Situations of escalating conflict are less humorous, but one still needs courage to put an end to them. Suppose a married couple is caught in a vicious circle: the man is always critical because his wife does not like him, and his wife does not like him because he is always critical. How can this vicious circle be broken? Each person justifies inappropriate behaviour by appealing to the inappropriate behaviour of the other person. Everyone is waiting for the other person to put an end to the inappropriate behaviour first. They may both wait for a long time, unless one of them makes an "advance of love". For example, the man could suddenly put an end to his criticism (even though his wife rejects him). Or the wife could begin to treat her husband with graciousness and respect (even though he is always critical). This changes the situation, because the reason for the inappropriate behaviour is removed for one of the parties. Why would the husband be critical when his wife is nice to him? Why would the wife reject her partner if he controls his behaviour? The vicious circle is broken. If both of them make an "advance of love", it collapses immediately.

Ahrendt: That requires a huge amount of trust – trust that something will change.

Lukas: Yes, it does. People who want to change the world must change *themselves*. Trust is necessary, but so is the awareness that we are free to make changes. And that every individual plays an important role in deciding which things will change, and whether for the better or the worse. Freedom is primarily the freedom to act responsibly or to choose not to.

Ahrendt: That sounds very different from what many people understand by freedom.

Lukas: Frankl taught us that freedom is never freedom *from* something (*from* our circumstances), but *for* something, namely to adopt a stance with respect to our circumstances, and to shape them creatively.

Ahrendt: But how is that freedom, if I cannot free myself from something, for example something unpleasant?

Lukas: Allow me to sketch a well-known logotherapeutic model for you. We can break down each concrete situation experienced by a given person into two parts. The left hand part we call the "domain of fate", the right hand part is the "space of personal freedom".

The domain of fate is defined as everything that is not (or is no longer) under the control of this person in this given life situation. This is admittedly a large domain. It includes the whole previous history of this person from the moment of his or her birth up until the present. None of this can be changed. This domain also includes the person's physical and psychic state as it now is. This can be changed in the future, but not in the present moment. It also includes everything that is decided either by other people, or by a transcendental fate that no one can grasp. It is an enormously large domain.

On the right hand side of the model is the space of personal freedom. What do we find there? After a bit of thought, it consists of two things: the behaviour and attitudes of the person in the here and now. The person can choose what to do and what not to do, and what inner attitudes will be adopted towards every detail of the domain of fate, as well as towards options for the future.

One of Frankl's most brilliant ideas was to reduce the whole of the enormous left hand side, the domain of fate, to "nothing", insofar as we can see it as the region in which we have no choice. Whereas on the small right hand side we have a galaxy of choices, from which we have the opportunity to pick out one of the "stars" and bring it to actualisation. This galaxy of stars is admittedly constrained. If someone is severely ill and bedridden, or in prison, that person's choices are restricted. Nevertheless, they exist – right up until the last breath of life.

Let us pursue this thought further. Are these stars in the galaxy which are available to us all equally valuable and worthy of being actualised? Is it a matter of indifference which one we choose? By no means! Our possible choices include completely stupid ones. We can jump off a balcony, we can dye our hair bright yellow and purple, and so on. We also have possible choices which are evil, as the newspapers report on a daily basis. *The art of life consists of identifying, selecting and realising the possibility that is most worthy of being actualised.* In the terminology of our model: to identify the brightest (= most meaningful) star in the galaxy of possibilities on the right hand side, and transfer it to the left hand side, to our life history, whereupon it becomes an abiding and inviolable truth about our self.

We should be clear about the fact that it is *possibilities* and not *actualisations* that disappear. Stars that are not chosen fade away. If I do not jump from the balcony, this possibility disappears from my present life. If I do jump, this possibility ceases to be a possibility and becomes (a tragic) part of reality. Together with all of its consequences, it becomes a part of my past, from which it can never be removed. Everything which is once chosen becomes eternal.

This model can be very helpful in logotherapeutic practice. Patients seek help because their domain of fate includes something bad that they cannot deal with. It may be a trauma, a tragedy, fears, conflicts, bad habits or depressive moods. A clear diagnosis is always necessary. But then we need to direct patients' attention to the domain of individual freedom and point out the galaxy of stars that exists in their present situation. To let them be surprised by the richness of possibilities that exists for them despite and in the midst of their darkness. And to invite them to reach out for their brightest star – to discover the best of all their possibilities. Logotherapy is not a psychotherapy of *uncovering*, but of *discovering*.

What must be discovered is the one thing in the here and now that will do good to the person and also in the world. Unfortunately this is not necessarily the most pleasurable or preferred option for the patient. Sometimes it is something that is very difficult to do. But, 1. it is always something that the patient *can* do (otherwise it would not be in their domain of freedom) and 2. it is always something that they *should* do, because it is in harmony with their conscience. Patients must always decide for themselves what they will do, but we can offer them help in putting it into practice, and we can honestly assure them that the darkness around them will grow lighter when they enrich their life with the light of the star that is worthy of being made real.

Ahrendt: Is the key question what is good for us and the world in a particular situation?

Lukas: One could put it like that. Frankl said, "Every deed is its own monument". This means that every action that is performed or omitted, but also every inner stance and attitude, is carved into our own monument, our own identity. Happy people are those who can live content with themselves. And one can only be content if one has a life filled with meaning.

Ahrendt: It sounds like we have an incredible responsibility for our own lives!

Lukas: For ourselves and the effect that we have. Frankl made the point well when he wrote in his book *The Doctor and the Soul*:

"...there is something fearful about man's responsibility. But at the same time something glorious! It is fearful to know that at this moment we bear the responsibility for the next, that every decision from the smallest to the largest is a decision for all eternity, that at every moment we bring to reality – or miss – a possibility that exists only for the particular moment." [1]

Ahrendt: Dr. Lukas, thank you very much for this instructive talk!

---

[1] Viktor E. Frankl, *The Doctor and the Soul*, New York, Vintage Books, 1986, p. 35.

Case Studies
from a Logotherapist's Practice
(Elisabeth Lukas und Heidi Schönfeld)

Introduction

Lukas: In 2005, as the controversial topic of active euthanasia was under debate, Jansen-van der Weide and Onwuteaka-Philipsen carried out a number of surveys in the Netherlands. One of the topics explored was the reasons given by sufferers of serious illness for seeking help to die.[2] The result was unexpected. Depression was a factor for only 7% of the respondents, and 30% of the respondents, less than a third, cited the fear of pain. The most common reason for wanting to die was the "futility of suffering", given by 67% of the respondents. This was closely followed by a fear of "degradation", in other words, a loss of dignity, mentioned by 65%. The researchers were astonished to find that most of the factors that rob seriously ill patients of a will to live cannot be addressed by medical treatment and palliative care alone.

I have mentioned this study because experience of healthy people or those who "merely" suffer from mental health disorders shows that their ability to affirm life fundamentally depends on the following two conditions: they need to be able to 1. see meaning in their life despite all their difficulties, and 2. be aware of their unconditional value and personal dignity. If either of these conditions is satisfied, there is a much greater inhibition threshold towards endangering one's own (or someone else's) life, sabotaging it, shortening it, or

---

[2] From: *Active Euthanasia – An Analysis*, master thesis by Maximilian Schlegel for the PPE course at the Ludwig-Maximilians-University Munich, p 16.

plunging into a whirl of instant gratification without considering the consequences. Responsible existence requires a horizon of meaning and values.

There is a field of psychotherapy that specialises in meaning and personal dignity, and this is the logotherapy of Viktor E. Frankl. It begins with the axiom that there is no situation in life, no matter how complicated, that does not offer the possibility of meaning, and that no human being, whether unborn, disabled, terminally ill or otherwise is without a human spirit that puts them on a spiritual level with all other human beings. Building on these principles, Frankl developed a system of psychotherapeutic concepts that offer a "psychotherapy with dignity" that is unique amongst the myriad treatment options that exist today. A number of poignant case studies reported by Heidi Schönfeld, which are reproduced in this book with my comments, bear witness to this.

What I myself was able to learn directly from Frankl in my training as a psychologist, I passed on by teaching others. Dr. Heidi Schönfeld is one of my former students; one of whom I am very proud. She continues faithfully in the tradition of Frankl's thought, which is why it is an honour for me to be admitted into her therapeutic practice in the following pages to look over her shoulder in her life-changing work. I am convinced that the readers of this book will also be fascinated to "look over her shoulder". If they are non-specialists, they will be able to use some of the healing methods for their own benefit. If they are specialists, they may be inspired to engage intensively with Frankl's specialist writings.

We live in times of great unrest and increased disorientation. To reflect on the essence what it means to be human, and to listen to the "inner voice" within us that knows and proclaims what is meaningful in every situation, gives us a spiritual grip that can carry us through any turbulence. It is impossible to prevent fate from raining blows down on us, whether as individuals or as whole communities, but *how we deal with them* is in our hands, and for us alone to decide.

Our dignity is rooted in this "ultimate freedom"; it is our task to make sensitive use of it in harmony with our values. If *this one thing* is remembered after reading this book, this more than justifies the collaborative efforts of my colleague and myself.

Dealing with Self-Pity

Lukas: There are a number of popular sayings that express how easy it is to focus on other people's mistakes – as through a magnifying glass – while one's mistakes are swept under the carpet. That is why you should "sweep in front of your own door first" and remove the "plank in your own eye" before the "speck in your brother's eye". The prevalence of sayings like this suggests that the idea has a long tradition. Although it conflicts with the widespread idea that well-being primarily involves taking care of oneself, many people have a habit of examining and complaining about the weaknesses and fail-ures of the people around them. This is probably not done out of genuine interest in other people, but in order to make oneself appear better by comparison, and so that the blame for one's own "reactive" weaknesses and failures can be gracefully shifted onto others.

There is a high price, however, for appearing better and less blameworthy. It is actually a double price. First, the hidden ethical yardstick of our personal conscience is difficult to fool. It flutters between faith and skepticism when we tell it about the villains all around us, who deserve nothing but resentment and rejection. It lets much unkindness pass without reproach, but it is never 100% con-vinced by our complaints and accusations. In its spiritual depths it senses that we are sweeping something under the carpet or ignoring the plank in our own eye, and it has to be violently hammered down for this sense to be driven away.

Second, the psychic effect of self-pity is to spread emptiness into one's own life like a cancer. A preoccupation with blaming other people, finding fault with their actions, reproaching them, and seeing their objectionable behaviour as the cause of one's own circumstances of existence, leaves few resources for determining one's own way of life. People who see themselves as a sacrifice to their circumstances allow themselves to be led like a lamb to the slaughter, rather than evading the blows of fate. Even in the absence of such blows, they wait and cower, wailing about the injustices of a world full of blows waiting to fall. How can they see that the world is full of opportunities and possibilities for meaning if they never even enter it?

We see cases of these kinds all the time in psychotherapeutic practice.[3] Whether it was a family member that first led them to the slaughterhouse, or whether they found their own way there for some distorted reason, they now cower there, waiting for the bad things that they expect to come. It requires considerable effort to encourage them to leave this place of immolation – which often exists only in their imagination.

Schönfeld: Mrs G, a 48-year-old patient, came to see me. She immediately let out a great succession of sighs: she can no longer cope with her life because "everyone" makes her life so difficult. "Everyone" means, above all, her family. Mrs G had approached a psychotherapist years ago for advice, but the discussions had not helped her at that time. Given *her* family, not even a therapist could have thought of anything helpful, she says. Who knows what the therapist said, but there is no need for this intemperate and unending complaint. So I try to limit the time I devote to her sense of injury. Self-pity is a quality that must not be allowed to grow wild, otherwise it suffocates like a creeper.

---

[3] The illnesses, concerns, and problems that we discuss in these chapters are equally likely to affect women or men.

Mrs G begins by describing her relationship with her father, which has become completely awful. She tells me that the 78-year-old gentleman has recently remarried and has hardly spoken to her since. He takes a lot of short trips with his adventurous wife. He has also updated his house and replaced the vegetable beds in the garden with flower beds. It certainly no longer looks like her family home as she knows it, now that his new wife has decorated everything so stylishly. When I ask how much Mrs G is still making contact with her father and his wife, she pours out a flood of criticism. "It wouldn't be any good now!" is the essence of this outburst. Her father doesn't care about her problems at all, he is no longer like a father to her. "My goodness," I think, "she is middle aged, he is an old man. How much more 'fatherhood' does she require from him?"

Mrs G complaints are not to be stopped, however: her whole family is so difficult. She only sees her younger brother a few times a year when he invites her to his children's birthday parties. They don't talk much, because the brother always has a lot to do, but at least they treat one another with respect. This contrasts with her relationship with her older sister, who has been jealous of her since she was a child. Her sister cannot stand to be criticised. She is overactive and highly involved in the city's art scene, which keeps her very busy. For years, she has had no time at all for Mrs G. For her birthday, she sent her a very pretty art postcard, but it only had the briefest of messages. She did not even call. When Mrs G wrote to her sister at Christmas two years ago to say how hurt she felt, she only got an angry email message in reply. Since then, Mrs G has completely cut off relations with her sister. So apart from seeing her brother at her nephews' birthday parties, she is completely alone.

Lukas: If you yourself feel stuck in an empty life, it takes enormous generosity to allow your loved ones and fellow human beings to enjoy lives full of meaningful projects! The difference is especially hard to accept when it comes to one's own family. This woman's father is cherishing his new wife, enjoying his travels, and creating a comfortable home for himself according to his own desires. In a bundle of misery like Mrs G, this may well cause envy to run high. Her brother is a good man, but blessed with children and other activities, and the sister has discovered a penchant for art and a community in which she can get involved and make a contribution. In the face of this, Mrs G has only bitterness and loneliness to offer. Like a child, she is secretly begging for a few crumbs of affection, to be heard in her grief, to be freed from the cocoon in which she has enclosed herself, but she only succeeds in scaring her entire family away. Everyone is clearly happy not to hear from her or see her very often, for no one knows how to help her, and everyone is made uncomfortable by her demands to participate in a happiness that is out of her reach.

When Viktor E. Frankl wrote about *noogenic neuroses* and *noogenic depression* in his books, he was addressing a category of patients who had not been covered by the textbooks of his time. They show no pronounced symptoms and are not characterised by any objective state of distress. Often they possess more than they need, living lives of material abundance. They often enjoy adequate physical fitness and a respectable education – or at least they *could* enjoy these things if they were able to enjoy anything. But they are not capable of enjoyment. Because nothing really matters to them. Nothing has any significance or meaning. And because "nothing matters" to them, this indifference carries over into their human relationships: they don't care about others, and others don't care about them. An "existential vacuum" (Frankl) engulfs them.

Some such patients rebel wildly against it and slide into a hectic struggle. They lurch from one short-term relationship to another, leading to more and more frustration. Some, on the other hand, give up and sink into chronic pessimism, in which they end or reject relationships in anticipation of failure, which guarantees that they fail repeatedly. One could feel great pity for them if they were not so intensely suffused with self-pity that one would almost rather let them wallow in their misery and spend one's pity on those who have suffered a more objectively measurable form of suffering.

The lack of sympathy they experience has its own reasons. Anyone who squanders sympathy readily accuses others of not offering enough sympathy. But accusing others of not having enough sympathy is a guaranteed way to lose all remaining sympathy.

Schönfeld: Mrs G says that she lived with a partner for years. This relationship was also not ideal. When she consulted a psychologist about it, she realised that her attachment to this man was purely selfish. She simply didn't want to be alone. This realisation struck her like a blow, because she did not want to be selfish. For this reason, she separated from her husband. Since then, she has had no close relations with another person.

The friendships she used to have with female friends have also broken down over the years. Her friends have been increasingly preoccupied with their own families and have had less and less interest in meeting up with Mrs G. Life is so hard when people treat you so badly – this is the ever-recurring refrain in Mrs G's account.

Lukas: It's time to end this refrain. My colleague was absolutely right to set a limit to her patient's complaints right from the very beginning, because there is a danger that she will become more and more mired in unproductive self-pity. Her statements are already bordering on the irrational. The discovery of selfish motives should not be a reason for separation, but rather for overcoming that recognised selfishness so that genuine love can grow. And far from distracting friends from their family duties, a true friend will support them in a compassionate way. My colleague will have to work hard to develop the patient's sense of responsibility and eventually (to use a popular phrase) to persuade her to clean up her own act.

Schönfeld: I invite Mrs G to answer a question. "If I raised my hand just now and struck you" – I carefully suggested this gesture – "what would my behaviour say about *you*? What could be deduced from this about *your* character?"

Mrs G stops short and thinks about this, but she can find no answer. Finally, she raises her shoulders and says, "I really don't know what this is supposed to say about *me*." I nod affirmatively, because she has understood the situation. "Exactly! If I struck you, it wouldn't say anything at all about *you*. What is interesting, however, is what would happen to *me* in that instant. The moment I do such a thing, I make myself a violent person – do I not?"

Mrs G is amazed, but after a little reflection she says: "Yes, that's true."

I give her a second example. "What would it say about *your* character if I secretly took your bag and stole your purse from it?" We readily agree that my theft would tell us absolutely nothing about *her* and *her* character. However, something would again happen to *me*, namely, I would become a thief. Behind these seemingly simple mental constructs lies a powerful principle: everything I do, everything that emanates from me into the world, shapes my character and writes the story about me into the truth. In my examples, it would have been *me* who would have been formed into a violent person or a thief in the case where I chose to commit a crime. It would not tell us anything about Mrs G. Only her response to my actions would reveal something about her. Because now it would be her turn. Would she fight back? Would she attack me? Would she run away? Would she protect herself? Would she talk to me? Would she remain silent? Would she cry? Would she remain calm? Now it is *her* turn to shape herself, and everything she does and everything that emanates from her will write *her* story into the truth. What will her story tell? Perhaps it will tell of prudence and bravery in the face of my wickedness, perhaps of brutal retaliation – there are many possibilities...

We discuss this principle for a long time and ponder it carefully. It cannot easily be dismissed. I carefully apply it to Mrs G's previous interpretations of her life. All of a sudden, what other people do or don't do is of little importance. Suddenly it is irrelevant whether or not her father pays attention to her. It doesn't matter if her sister annoyed her with an angry email message. It matters little what emanates from others, for this shapes only themselves. What is interesting for Mrs G is the story of her *own* past actions – and from this point of view, the evidence in her own life turns out to be rather dismal. Nevertheless, from this perspective, we can spell out one event in her life after another in a completely new way. The result is that Mrs G is not exactly proud of our findings, but acquires a greater and greater conviction that this should all change. From now on, she wants to be able to be proud of the person that she herself decides should radiate into the world from her.

Lukas: My colleague has certainly given her patient a brilliant logotherapeutic lesson! She clearly managed to balance the emotional fluctuations between amazement, insight, shock, and embarrassment in Mrs G so skilfully that the insight outweighed the embarrassment. The entire course of the conversation is remarkable! Here a woman, who incessantly complains about the people around her, abruptly discontinues her complaints and accusations, focusses her attention on a serious matter, understands the essential point of a difficult principle, allows it to be applied to her own life and agrees to change. It is almost a miracle: it is as if her scales fell from her eyes – and all self-pity from her soul. I can only congratulate my colleague.

The patient had said one thing that seems like it could be therapeutically useful. This was when she said she didn't want to be selfish. Whether this was sincere or not, the intention sounded promising. Now she says that she wants to be proud of her own actions and responses in the future. This is good, intentions like this fill up an inner emptiness, an "existential vacuum". It must only be ensured that these intentions are of good quality and have sufficient force to be implemented. This is something that will have to be worked on in therapy.

Schönfeld: In the next session, Mrs G asks whether there is a general criterion to decide what one can justifiably be proud of. I suggest a thought by Viktor Frankl. Frankl suggests that we are on the right track if we orient our actions towards meaning. This sounds convincing, but it is not as simple as it may seem at first. What does it mean in practice to "act meaningfully"? If one were to conduct a survey, many people would spontaneously answer: "What is meaningful to me is what is to my advantage." This is not completely wrong, but I explain to my patient that it is not enough. A head of state could come up with the idea that it would be to his advantage to possess the oil wells or ore deposits in the neighbouring country and it would therefore be meaningful to invade this neighbouring country. Would that really be meaningful? Mrs G immediately realises that it can't be meaningful to harm someone. We agree: what is meaningful is always the best possible thing for *everyone* involved.

We think about the idea of "best possible" for a while. Is there a "best possible" thing to choose in every situation in life? Certainly! Provided that one can choose at all and is not, for example, an infant, asleep, comatose, or confused, possibilities always fan out before us, and amongst them is one that, under the given circumstances, ranges between "optimal" and "tolerable" for everyone concerned, depending on how the circumstances are arranged. It may not be an act of heroism that meaning demands of us. It may be something completely banal, for example, to cook lunch. Why not? But it can also be something more difficult, for example, to go without lunch if you are severely overweight. Mrs G is amazed: *as long as we are conscious, there is always a "best possible", and if we decide to do it – whether it is easy or difficult to implement – we can be satisfied with ourselves.* She has never seen it that way before.

I return to Mrs G's initial complaint about her sister's indignant reaction to the letter that she wrote to her two years ago. We do not know why the sister was so outraged at the time, and speculating about this is not useful. Maybe she just wrote the email precipitately when she was in a hurry. Or maybe it was a kind of reflex action, because something had hit a sensitive nerve. Best to let it rest. What we do know, however, is that Mrs G has been icily silent since her sister's abrupt rejection. This iciness has also affected her own life, she admits. "But how should I have responded?" she says in her defence.

I invite her to think again about Frankl's thesis. There is a "best possible" for everyone involved. Mrs G looks skeptical at first, but I play out various alternatives with her in retrospect. She could have spoken her mind in an equally aggressive email in reply to her sister (she had done so quite often in her thoughts). She could have complained to her brother and tried to get him to take her side. She could have shared her sister's angry message with her art friends to show them how callously her sister treats her relatives. Her "space of revenge" would also include other possibilities, but all of them would have inflicted more damage, and this contradicts the criterion of meaning!

What other possibilities would have existed? Mrs G suggests that she could have explained to her sister why she felt so hurt by her attack. Not bad! "Could you also turn that around?" Perhaps my patient could have asked her sister what upset *her* so much that she used such harsh words? Mrs G agrees that this would have been a constructive question. She could have written back that she wanted to meet and talk in person about their misunderstandings. How would her sister have reacted to this? "Favourably, I expect," says Mrs G. "My sister would certainly have been willing to meet me. But I would have had to overcome a big inner hurdle to be able to tell her, 'Something is not right with our relationship, let's see if we can fix it!' I don't think I could have done that then in my moment of rage!" "Oh yes," I replied, "you can do much more than you think. To be proud of yourself, you have to do something remarkable..." "I know that now," says Mrs G with a smile, "but nobody told me that back then".

Lukas: Frankl called the procedure used by my colleague an *awareness extension*. People afflicted with psychic disorders often suffer from the opposite: a narrowing of their field of awareness. This awareness does not relate to physical vision, but to an "inner vision". In the face of strong affective pressure, they often see very few ways, or even only one way in which they can behave. They are almost completely unaware of any alternatives. In such cases, one of the main tasks of the therapist is to make the patient aware of the wide range of possibilities that are still available, even in the midst of an emotional crisis. This is, for example, the best way to encourage more positive behaviour in criminal offenders. A person who has hitherto been stuck on a one-way street – getting angry means pulling out a knife – learns that this is in fact a crossroads from which numerous paths branch off. Symbolically, the anger lies in the middle of the crossroads, and the angry person can circle around it and look down any of the branching streets. There is a "Knife Road", an "Argument Road", a "Humor Road", an "Apology Road", an "Understanding Road", a "Doesn't Matter Road", and so on. It is already a big step forward if the person concerned reads these street signs, because this confronts the person directly with his or her freedom to choose how to deal with the anger, instead of being passively driven towards a "dead end".

In noogenic neuroses and depressions we find similar clusters of one-way streets, with or without criminal impulses. The combination of an empty life with self-pity and complaint is extremely common. In my experience, it takes a lot of effort to make the place on the crossroads palatable to such patients, because they are used to blaming their problems on everyone else, much as criminal offenders often do. That these patients are more peaceable than such offenders is attributable more to inertia and indifference of spirit than to a more developed ethical sense.

With Mrs G, however, it has been possible to initiate her into "reading street names". We have also achieved something beyond this! Soon she is able to reject dingy dead ends and find a regal high street. An enormous therapeutic success. Will she dare to go down this street? The light is green.

At this point, let me add two theoretical remarks.

1. What allows us as humans to respond to our circumstances in many different possible ways is our ability to self-distance (Frankl). We can move away from ourselves in spirit, and look back at ourselves from the distance we have gained. In this way, all our waves of emotion become visible as they are from outside, and only from this place of external observation can they be controlled. Sometimes a dialogue with ourselves can make things clearer. For example, if Mrs G were to say to herself, "you are disappointed in your father," or "you are sad about your loneliness," she would cease to identify herself with her disappointment or grief; these would become unwelcome companions who might ensnare her, but whom she could overcome. She could then, turning to herself, continue: "Well, my father can amuse himself! Go find yourself a hobby, then you'll enjoy yourself as well!"or "What do you want exactly? You still have half your life ahead of you! Save your grief for a serious crisis and do something!"

The excellent advice that one has freely and readily available for other people, can be calmly given to and heeded by oneself.

My teacher, Viktor E. Frankl, said that during the Second World War, in the middle of the hell of a concentration camp, he imagined himself standing at the lectern of a brightly lit, warm lecture hall giving a talk about dealing with trauma. In this way, he was able to distance himself from his current pain and apply to himself all the tricks of trauma management that he had just described to his imaginary audience.

2. Mrs G was trained to explore the best (for everyone) of all the possibilities available to her. This is what a "pure search for meaning" looks like. The key question is always this: what is really the best? A suitable yardstick that we can apply is the *expected development of the current situation.* If we choose a given possibility, will it tend to lead towards a positive or a negative outcome? This is why, in the conversation with the patient described above, my colleague checked how the patient's sister would have taken the possible course of action retrospectively imagined by Mrs G, namely an offer to set aside their mutual animosity. Mrs G imagined that this would have led to a positive development in her relationship with her sister. Therefore, to have chosen this possibility would have been meaningful.

Unfortunately, predictions of this kind sometimes turn out to be false. Since we are not clairvoyant, we can never be sure that the outcomes we predict will in fact occur. Meaning in human life – as we intend to grasp it – can only be fulfilled "to the best of our knowledge and conscience," and can unexpectedly turn into something meaningless that we did not wish for. This does not absolve us from the obligation to search for meaning and act according to the meaning we understand, because we have no more reliable yardstick to apply.

One of the biggest problems for the dawning epoch in human history that predictability is declining in many areas of life and science. As the number of possible actions increases, it becomes increasingly difficult to predict the consequences of any given action. We can manipulate genes and atoms, we can program robots with intelligence and the ability to learn, we can control the forces of nature...but we can't know where exactly all of this will lead. *Decreasing predictability complicates the search for meaning,* and not only in our lives as individuals. Generations yet to come will have to work hard to develop yet further their "meaning organ" of conscience (Frankl) in order to meet the challenges of their time.

Schönfeld: We continue to discuss the disastrous interaction between Mrs G and her sister. Is it still going on? Mrs G says that the last two years have been filled with resentment. The icy silence between the two of them has not yet thawed. What could she do but leave things as they are? After all, the sister could also get in touch with her!

Careful – this relapse must be addressed right away! What others do tells us about *them*, but that is only of secondary relevance for Mrs G. She wants to change *her* nature, so the important question is what action by *Mrs G* would enable her to pat herself on the shoulder, something that she might even be proud of in the future! We ponder this question for a while. Mrs G hesitantly explores the idea that she could send out an invitation to a family meeting where everyone could talk. Perhaps the café in the neighboring town would be a suitable place for this meeting, because there is a pedestrian zone nearby that is a nice place to walk and chat. This sounds good to me. But Mrs G hesitates and admits that quarrels could very easily flare up again. She thinks of her father with his new partner and the three siblings suddenly sitting at a table opposite each other after having lived apart for so long. This needs to be considered too. Mrs G slowly warms up to playing the role of peacemaker, but idea of the café seems risky to her. She wants to think this idea through in detail until our next therapy session.

Weeks later, Mrs G tells me what she has thought about in the meantime. She is sure about one thing: it is time for her family's ice age to end. Mrs G is really tired of it and the others probably are as well. It would be very noble of her to invite her sister to her home, but if she is honest, something in her resists this idea. She is afraid that her sister might brutally or summarily reject her invitation. And what if she comes, but the conversation degenerates once again into a shower of accusations? She still carries so much resentment that the encounter would be a minefield.

Mrs G therefore has to come up with something less risky. In summer there is usually a summer festival in their church community. This time, a group of young people will stage a play they have written as a fundraiser for setting up a new youth centre. This would be a good opportunity for Mrs G to invite her whole family. The invitation would be *her* initiative, but in the context of the community event, it would be impersonal enough that old antagonisms would not immediately be aroused. They would watch the play together, the ticket cost would be for a good cause, and they wouldn't have to start a personal conversation right away. Her brother's children would be there, which could provide a distraction at critical moments. There would be a barbecue stand and some salads, so they could talk about the play over some food and bond a bit. It would be an encounter with an open outcome, but at least the estranged family members would meet again.

I am thrilled. It is impressive how sensitive my patient can be, and how ready she is to be self-overcoming; who would have expected this? In pursuing a possibility for meaning, there is no way of ruling out a disaster. Anyone who keeps it firmly in view, however, will be able to overcome the disaster if it occurs. I discuss with Mrs G some details about the invitation process and a few contingency plans, but I have no reservations about her project.

Lukas: Mrs G's therapy is "running like clockwork". However, I am afraid that that there is still a lot of work to do. Bringing peace to the family is undoubtedly an important goal, even a primary goal, but it will not eliminate the existential vacuum that has appeared in Mrs

G's life. Even if her life includes more frequent and more agreeable interactions with her relatives in the future – which is not guaranteed even in times of peace – Mrs G cannot depend on her family and share their preferences. In order to catch an "existential upwind", she will have to develop initiatives that correspond to her own nature and are productive beyond that nature.

Although she doesn't notice it, Mrs G lives under extremely favourable circumstances. She has everything she needs. She does not have to starve, freeze, or perish in case of illness, and she can afford many small extravagances. Every day she can prepare herself a delicious breakfast and enjoy the smell of fresh coffee in her kitchen. She can read, hear, walk, clothe herself, bend down, and do so much more that masses of underprivileged people, for various reasons, cannot. Just 200 years ago, she would have been on the verge of becoming an elderly woman at the age of 48, whereas today she is in the category of middle-aged women who often start a new qualification, try out a new relationship, take on a new area of responsibility or explore distant parts of the world by plane, ship or coach. She has so much, but she lacks the awareness of what she has, which my colleague will help her to acquire. Nothing can be taken for granted! Nothing should be undervalued!

And no one should turn up their nose at a personal hobby. Of course, there may not be room for it in a life which is already overstrained with obligations, with a daily calendar crowded with appointments. But if there is enough time for it, a hobby can be a blessing. Even with children it is a good idea to encourage them to find a suitable way of exercising their talents outside of school. They will benefit from it later. A hobby provides an excellent balance to the necessity of work, which can be monotonous or unwanted. Hobbies bring colour and variety into daily life and can even serve as a refuge into which one can retreat in the face of worries and difficulties. They prevent one from churning around in what is unpleasant and sticking to it mentally and emotionally.

Hobbies do much more than to fill the gaps in a life filled with emptiness. They increase spiritual flexibility, as one enters their domain, focuses on them, and leaves this domain again to devote oneself to one's usual concerns. They also stimulate intellectual growth, because a hobby usually expands the range of skills of the person who practices it. *Summa summarum* a hobby educates one to devoted activity and protects one from stagnation; what more could Mrs G want?

Schönfeld: It may be a few months until the summer gathering, but my patient is satisfied with her decision. *She* will be the one who will work towards the resolution of the family situation, no matter what the others make of it. Then she will have done her best for the family relationships. A sore point in her life has begun to heal.

Behind it, a wound has emerged that was previously hidden: there is too much boredom in her life. She works as a secretary in a large company and does not find her job very exciting, but she is glad that at least the weekdays are busy. She has not made any close friends at work, although she occasionally has a brief exchange of ideas with her colleagues. In the evenings she makes herself some dinner, does a few household jobs and watches TV until bedtime. Weekends and holidays, which should be a highlight, are a sensitive topic. As she's been living alone since her relationship broke down, she has too much time that she doesn't know how to use. Cleaning, shopping, cooking, watching TV, that's not enough make a fulfilling life. Before I can object, she waves me aside. I'm not to suggest occupational therapy. Well-meaning acquaintances have given her enough of that. That isn't for her!

Smiling, I take a piece of paper and draw (copying a model by Elisabeth Lukas) two hemispheres placed one above the other. One hemisphere is meant to symbolise that there is a lot of need around us. Our world moans and groans, and on all sides and in every corner there is a need for hands to take hold of, and hearts to relieve distress. This can take the form of small things that are helpful, such as a kind greeting or a word of comfort, all the way up to a major commitment, for example to a community project. The other hemisphere is a bowl with the individual talents of a single person – here the talents of Mrs G. In this bowl lies everything that she can do well; all the abilities that she has acquired and developed from childhood. This is the domain of her personal competence. First we look at this second hemisphere together. What are Mrs G's strengths?

My patient has hardly ever thought about this. She feels her way forward slowly. She thinks she is a good listener. But people often take advantage of this and burden her with accounts of their problems, which is annoying to her. She prefers it when she can talk about her won problems I have to slow her down before she misses the point. We are looking for *your* strengths. Well, she has an acute aesthetic sensibility, she can make beautiful things out of colours and shapes. Also, she can write well and type quickly. This is what her profession has taught her. Gradually we discover that religion plays an important role in her life. She would be willing to perform small services for others, such as shopping for someone with a disability, but she knows no one who needs this.

Her information is rather sparse, so we turn to the second hemisphere. This contains the many needs outside or beyond ourselves, needs which can only be met by a person with the right qualities. We try hard to ascertain where in the environment of Mrs G we could find such a need. There would be a need for someone to help immigrants find their way to government offices. In the city there are some retirement homes that would gladly welcome visitors for elderly residents. There is a shortage of volunteers all over the place. Young working mothers would be happy to "rent" a grandmother by the hour. Mrs G becomes increasingly animated. There are many community and church events. Who decorates the tables, arranges the flowers, designs the invitation cards? Did she not say that she has an aesthetic sensibility? And as for her writing skills, well, if elderly residents in a retirement home would dictate their memoirs, she could write these stories up and present them in attractive folders. Mrs G is becoming even more excited and alert. A side of the world is opening up before her that she has never noticed before. A side that is full of attractive tasks and projects. I ask her where there is a really pressing need. She does not know – she knows that there is a shortage of carers for people with dementia, but she cannot imagine herself performing this kind of service.

Finally, we agree that she will take long walks in her free time in the coming weeks. She should let her thoughts wander around the two hemispheres, which are longing to unite into a smooth, luminous sphere. "What talents do I have? What do I do well and enjoy doing?" And: "Where is there a need for someone who can do exactly this thing well and enjoy doing it?" If the two hemispheres can be matched, both will be in a much better state than before.

Lukas: It is a pleasure to see how my colleague took up a theoretical model of mine and cleverly integrated it into the therapeutic process. She actually succeeded in eliciting a few first self-transcendent steps from the egocentric patient. Nevertheless, I hesitate to give too optimistic an assessment of Mrs G's search for meaning thus far. My reason is that it is focused too much on social activities, whereas Mrs G, in my opinion, has poor social skills.

Experience with patients suffering from neuroses shows that they tend to overestimate their social skills. They often dream of "helping others" even as they are constantly annoying others. They are normally weak when it comes to cooperation. This is especially true for Mrs G. Not only has she fallen out with all her relatives. Her relationship has capsized. She has denounced every therapist who has tried to treat her. She brushes off all the well-meaning acquaintances who advise her to find something to do with herself. She has no friends at work, and if anyone wants to confide in her, she is uncomfortable listening to their problems. I would advise Mrs G not to volunteer in the community.

That doesn't mean she has no talents. But until the "first hemisphere" is thoroughly inspected, and Mrs G's true strengths are thoroughly explored, no vision will crystallise that could fit into the "second hemisphere". Nevertheless, this logotherapeutic help has sown enough fertile seed that one has good reason to hope that it will grow sooner or later.

Schönfeld: We meet again after a few weeks, but unfortunately there has been no breakthrough yet. Nevertheless, Mrs G has discovered that she is interested in many things, even if her interests are apparently not needed by anyone. And the regular walks are much better than sitting in front of the TV, as she herself admits. Very well. I am not disappointed, because Mrs G's conversation has already changed significantly from our first sessions together. She no longer whines, she is no longer suffocating in self-pity, and she no longer complains about other people. Suddenly I stop. During one of her walks, Mrs G came across a poster announcing that there will be summer Promenade concerts beginning in the neighboring town in May. I am amazed, because she tells me this with such animation. In years gone by, she had been to these concerts many times, and it had been a great experience every time! "Why?" I ask. "Music is so wonderful!" she raves. She loves both classical works and modern gospel concerts. Now we just have to avoid losing the thread! I follow it up carefully by asking if she would like to be involved with actively singing instead of just listening. She had never thought about that. She has never sung anything since she was in the school choir. But...the room is silent for a minute. But...well, she has a good voice, she says. She can hit a note correctly, and she can sight read from a sheet of music. If a new song is taught in a church service, she finds it easy to learn.

We consider the subject from all sides, weigh up the pros and cons – but there are no cons in sight. Mrs G's enthusiasm mounts: Yes, she would very much like to sing in a choir! Now she needs some creativity. She needs to find out which amateur choirs exist in her area, when the auditions are, what admission criteria there may be, whether any new singers are needed. We look beyond her boundaries: if she has a good voice, she has something to give to the world. Music gives light to the world! Singing does not just give pleasure to the singers – it gives pleasure to *an audience*! Mrs G beams. Of course, she will energetically pursue this idea. She will start with her local church and then inquire about choirs everywhere. She may even contact the promenade choir, which she has only ever admired as a listener.

Mrs G leaves my practice full of excitement and anticipation for her new hobby, which – now she thinks about it – would have always been right for her. I wish her good luck. It will be a while until her family is invited to the summer gathering, but she has planned everything carefully. Nevertheless, I am not under any illusions. There will be more difficult days for Mrs G. Even if she finds fulfilment in a choir, there remain empty spaces left in her life that need to be filled. Mrs G is aware of this, because she takes the picture with the two hemispheres with her as she says goodbye and explains in a resolute voice: "I am only 48 years old and I do not want to live the life of a pensioner. I want to take hold of my future."

I wish her good luck with all my heart!

Dealing with Lovesickness

Lukas: There are a few statements by Viktor E. Frankl that sound extremely provocative. Only when you delve deeper into the accompanying explanations do you understand their meaning. One of these statements is Frankl's assertion that there is and can be no "unhappy love". In the course of life, almost every human being suffers from heartache at some point – languishes, longs for a response to overpowering feelings, and believes that the world will end if no response is forthcoming. The entanglements of love are at the centre of all cinematic thrillers and theatrical dramas, whether they take the form of wild jealousy, bitter rejection, forelorn affection or shameful deceit.

So how did Frankl justify his bold assertion that love and unhappiness cannot go together? Well, this depends on his understanding of love. If a person is "lovesick" in this sense, then this can be attributed to a "sick" understanding of love. To love does *not* mean that the beloved person satisfies the lover's desires. It does not mean that he or she is always there, caring for, understanding, comforting, or always helping him or her. It does not mean that he or she is always faithful or stays there unconditionally. It would be nice if it were so, it might even be so, but it is not to be *expected*. The first of Frankl's lessons on love is thus that *love does not expect anything.* True love wants nothing *from* the other person. It wants the very best for the other person. It wants to contribute to this "very best" to the best of its ability.

But how will it work out what is best for the other person? Well, that is a tricky question. When I think back to the years I worked in educational counselling, I still shudder about some parents who greatly harassed their children because they wanted the very best for them. But was that really what they wanted? Or did these parents want children they could boast about and successes they could count as their own? It was often a difficult struggle to communicate to parents like this what their children really needed and what was really good for them. *Love is not about oneself*, is the second of Frank's lessons on love. It is about *the beloved*. But to go back to the question, how can love know what is the best thing for the beloved? The following is what Frankl had to say about this: "Love enormously increases receptivity to the fullness of values. The gates to the whole universe of values are, as it were, thrown open."[4]

This coincides with the subjective experience of people in love, who suddenly see everything around them in a brighter light. They assess their personal circumstances and their future more positively and are generally more value-sensitive than they were before. Their growing appreciation of values causes them to recognize the most wonderful inner qualities in their beloved, and with amazing intuition they sense what could unfold from the wonderful things that are still latent in them. *Love sensitises one to possibilities for value*; this is the third of Frank's lessons on love. It sensitises one especially to the valuable possibilities of the *beloved person*. This does not mean that the other is covered in glory. A total idealisation of the beloved being is more likely to be a stunted "love" which is focussed on the self and wants to set the self up with a brilliant match. True love, according to Frankl, involves both a realistic recognition of the beloved as they are *and* a vision of their very own ideal possibilities.

With this understanding of love we approach the aspect that by definition love can only enrich. As we have seen, it opens up a universe of values to the lover. This exhilarates the soul. It lets one anticipate the very best *in another and for the other*. It motivates one to want exactly this. It is this good will alone (and no pressure or pushing or forcing!) that motivates the other person to actualise it... and what if the other person does not do so? And if the other person does

---

[4] Viktor E. Frankl, The Doctor and the Soul, New York, Vintage Books, 1986, p. 133.

not appreciate the offered love or renounces it? *The treasure of love remains untouched*, that is the fourth of Frankl's lessons on love. A person has stretched out his or her spiritual antennae. Latent possibilities have been discovered. An exhilirating feeling has been enjoyed. The horizon of existence has been expanded. Perhaps the horizon of possession has diminished, but one does not "possess", or own, any human being, even a loved one. How wisely Erich Fromm said it: "Who am I, if I am what I have – and lose what I have?"[5] Only if you define yourself by what you have, need you and will you be unhappy if you lose your possessions.

Schönfeld: An emergency call comes in: the caller is crying so hard that I can hardly understand him. Only slowly does it become clear what it is all about. Mr H, in his mid-30s, is desperate. Through his halting words and profuse weeping the following picture emerges after much enquiry:

Seven weeks ago, his partner Susanne separated from him. This is the worst thing he has ever experienced. She was his first "real" girl-friend – by "real" he means that there were women before her in his life, but never before has he loved the way he loved Susanne. She has been the most important person in his whole life so far. Now he is completely devastated. He can no longer work, although his boss energetically exhorts him to do so. The young man works in the insurance industry; and a teary-eyed insurance consultant is no good to his customers. For weeks, his doctor has signed him off work and prescribed him antidepressants, but that hasn't helped at all. The young man cries his eyes out, sleeps very little, a maximum of two hours at a time, he says, and doesn't know how to go on.

The last seven weeks have been a plunge bath of misery. He has encountered Susanne occasionally. She has hugged and kissed him,

---

[5] Erich Fromm, Die Seele des Menschen. Ihre Fähigkeit zum Guten und zum Bösen, dtv, Munich, [2]1988, p. 53.

and then sent him on his way. His life is a complete disaster. The only bearable thing is that he does is to go to the gym for hours every day to exercise on the treadmill until he is exhausted. Physical exhaustion decreases his psychic pain a little.

After Susanne kicked him out of her apartment, he had to beg his parents to let him move back in with them. He didn't know where else to go. His parents were not very enthusiastic about this, because he had almost completely ignored them in recent years. He suddenly realised that he no longer has any close friends, because for the past three years he has only been involved with Susanne and her family and he has neglected everyone else. So his parents were not too pleased to see him, but they nevertheless offered him the use of his sister's room, as she had recently moved out.

The young man says he has lost everything: his friends, the woman for whom he "would have done anything", and her family, which had become his own family. What was especially cruel was that he had to give away his dog. Susanne had given him a labrador retriever, a small puppy. The animal had been affectionate and he had become very fond of it. Every day after work, sometimes with Susanne, but mostly alone, he had taken the dog for long walks. He had looked forward every day to seeing his dog. When he broke up with Susanne, however, he had to give the dog up that very day, because his parents were unwilling to have such a big animal in their relatively small rented apartment. He had no choice but to leave the dog with Susanne, who gave it away as soon as he left. He has no idea where the dog is now.

Lukas: Allow me a few rebellious comments as a specialist before I examine the patient's situation. Even a doctor's receptionist would have recognised right away from an emergency call like this that we are dealing with a *reactive depression*. The young man has experienced a painful event and is very unhappy about it. Absolutely *nothing* suggests that he suffers from a neurologically-based endogenous depression. To give just one example: in the case of depression of somatic origin, he would not have been able to work out for hours in a gym. So why prescribe antidepressants? Antidepressants regulate neurotransmitter production at the nerve synapses, but they do not erase suffering. A person has to deal with the suffering they experience with alertness of spirit and philosophical or religious sincerity; everything else misses the real problem. Clearly the doctor's prescription is of no use to Mr H. Yes, he sleeps too little. This, however, is an ambiguous symptom. Both endogenous and reactive depressions cause poor sleep – for different reasons. Even people without depression sometimes have disturbed sleep, and the reasons for this may be either grave or harmless. In any case, a severe loss, such as the one that Mr H has suffered, is serious enough to explain his lack of sleep (without our having to diagnose a psychotic illness).

As understandable as Mr H's reactive depression is, the question that nevertheless arises is: *Which aspects of this crisis* have caused him to slide from a natural reaction of grief into a reactive depression? There are many things that stand out in his report, which I would like to summarise, on the assumption that he is still quite immature in character despite his 30 years or so of age. His understanding of love certainly also differs from Frankl's. This is precisely where my colleague will start, hoping to correct Mr H's understanding of love in order to help him let go of Susanne in love and say goodbye to her in an amicable spirit. However, it seems to me that there are further areas in which Mr H may need some therapeutic assistance.

Maturity of character is essentially demonstrated by the fact that, after conscientious deliberation, one makes decisions independently, acts accordingly, and assumes responsibility for one's actions. There is no trace of this in Mr H's complaint. He is drowning not only in tears, but also in self-pity. *Others* think ill of him, according to his account, and he is the *poor victim*. Susanne rejects him cruelly, his parents are none too pleased at his crawling back to them and they refuse to take in his beloved dog, his boss demands better work performance, his doctor offers no suitable medication... and Mr H himself? He doesn't know where to go, he doesn't know what to do – but stop: he should know something by now! He knows that he has neglected his family and friends in recent years. Bravo, this insight has already made his grief worthwhile. It is high time that Mr H admits *his own contribution to his misfortune* and learns a lesson from it for the future.

Schönfeld: We make an appointment for him to come to my practice. When he comes to me, Mr H repeats his tragic account of how he has lost everything: his beloved, his dog, his friends; everything is gone. He sits in his younger sister's bedroom, can't face going to work, hardly sleeps, broods incessantly and cries more than ever before in his life. No, he doesn't intend to commit suicide, but he doesn't know how he can go on. What plunges him into even deeper misery is when Susanne calls or sends him text messages; always with a friendly tone, but always with the conclusion that a relationship with him is no longer possible. He thinks he's going crazy.

I let him know that I can understand him. No one can bear a constant oscillation between hope and disappointment, between "maybe" and "definitely not". To spend seven weeks in limbo is crushing. Although his state is extreme, it is "quite normal" for him to be sleeping badly. We spend some time discussing this idea of relative normality in the face of an abnormal situation and he comes to a remarkable conclusion: *if he does not let Susanne go in his heart, he will not be able to get back on his feet.*

Lukas: First of all, if a patient denies having suicidal intentions, this unfortunately doesn't tell us very much. Suicidal people almost always deny their suicidal intentions. This is why I never directly asked my patients about such intentions. If I feared for their affirmation of life, I followed Frankl's advice and asked them *why and what* *they still wanted to live for.* If they could spontaneously give me a "reason to live", I took this as a good sign. If they were at a loss, or muttered generalities, my concern for them increased. I have my doubts about whether Mr H could have described a "reason to live" at the time of this conversation. If a person thinks he or she has lost "everything", there is usually at some risk of suicide (and Mr H would not be the first to commit suicide out of heartbreak). Of course, what he believes is not real, because in fact Mr H has plenty of resources at his disposal. He is young, physically trained, and healthy. He has a level of education and vocational training that no one can take away from him, he is no orphan and can call on parents in times of need, he has not been fired from his job despite weeks of absence, he lives in a peaceful and wealthy country, and so on. There are millions of people on earth who have lost more than he has, but he is unable to see this. People who think only of themselves cannot see beyond their own horizons.

I would also like to highlight a second point. In therapeutic practice, it is a matter of principle not to speculate about people one does not know personally. This is why my colleague made no comments about Susanne. However, as an outsider, I can suggest a thought. By presenting himself as such a sorry figure, Mr H confronts Susanne with a proper dilemma. She wants to break up with him, but she probably doesn't want to be responsible for his breaking down. After all, the two have been close, and Susanne cannot help but empathise with Mr H's desolation, which has been caused by her desire for them to separate. So she is uneasy. She offers friendly gestures to minimise his pain, but on the other hand she does not want to create any misunderstanding. This is a mistake: her inconsistent behaviour does not relieve his pain at all, but stokes it up even more.

People make mistakes. Mr H fails to appreciate his many resources. Susanne is wrong about the best way to deal with her ex. *Errare humanum est...*

59

Schönfeld: We check exactly what Susanne wishes to convey. There are mixed messages coming from her, but the main message is always a firm no. She does not want to continue her relationship with Mr H. "I'm supposed to disappear from her life," he sobs bitterly. I do not intend to criticise his girlfriend's behaviour (which is largely understandable), but rather to try to refine his feelings for her. If he really loves her, then his love wants *her to be ok* – doesn't it? Yes, of course. If she thinks she is better off without him, what does his love have to say about this? Can it say, "If you feel better off without me, I will accept this and let you go"? He is silent for a long time. He thinks. That would actually be the most appropriate response – wouldn't it? Yes, of course. I admit that this is the hardest thing that can be expected from a loving person, but at the same time it is an immense triumph of love. It something done purely for the love of the other person.

We talk further about the phenomenon of love, and Mr H explains huskily that the three years together with Susanne were happiest time in his life so far. Well then, it is only logical that his grief now should be just as great. He should not complain, but should see his grief as a seal on the fact that these three years were not lived in vain, but were precious enough to be worth the experience. If the whole affair had been just a trivial affair in his eyes, he would not have to suffer now. That's true, he replies, but it hurts so much! How will he ever recover from this blow?

Mr H has not noticed, but at this point in our conversation he has reached an important turning point. 1. He has realized that his sincere affection for Susanne requires him to let her go for love, and 2. he has realized that his relationship with her was something beautiful and valuable that he would not want to have missed out on, even though it has now ended. This loosens his pathological fixation on Susanne and his time with her and allows him to concentrate on the present again, which he had lost sight of before. The question of *how he can recover from this blow of fate and the necessary renunciation of love* is a legitimate and important one, and this begins a new chapter in our reflection together.

Lukas: Aha, my colleague moves on to the other "construction sites" in Mr H's growth process. This does not put an end to the Susanne problem. It will continue to be under a process for a long time to come. But the focus of the problem management will gradually shift, and, if it is successful, it will improve Mr H's maturity. This may one day enable him to have a harmonious relationship not characterised by emotional dependence and bondage.

Here are a few psychological observations on the topic of emotions.

1. It makes a difference whether you lose a loved one through death or by voluntary departure. The grief is similar in strength, but there is a greater chance that the grief will be mixed with feelings of anger and rage when a loved one leaves by choice. Often love – or that which is thought to be love – turns into hate. One could see hate as a continuation of the former bond of love, but with the opposite sign. The hater will not let go of the hated person. The hater is tragically tied to the object of hate and condemned constantly to relive memories of him or her. Hate is *not* the opposite of love, but a perverted form of love (which has never actually been true love for the other, but something more self-centred right from the beginning). The opposite of love is indifference.

2. Anger and rage have the potential to feed on themselves. They begin with a feeling of upset and disappointment that can still be reined in. But then, ever-circling thoughts weave a murky web around them. These thoughts, the "Why?" and "Why do I deserve this?" and "How could they do this to me?" considerably increase the negative intensity of the feelings. The anger and rage mount. This is how they can lead to surprisingly disproportionate outbursts of aggression, which are perceived by other people as

complete overreactions. Other people know the reasons behind the upset and disappointment, but they know nothing of the web of thought that has been woven over them.

3. A temporary *targeted mental distraction* is recommended as a response to initial feelings of upset and disappointment, in order to dampen the self-reinforcing tendency of these feelings. Thoughts should not be allowed to circle round and round the source of the pain. Mr H reported that he was able to "switch off" on the treadmill. Great! Taking a deep breath, going for a walk, reading, playing music, drawing, coding, cooking, cleaning, visiting museums Any activities that are more "active" than "passive" help with maintaining self-control. If upset and disappointment are not fuelled by thought, they do not fan themselves into roaring fires that burn away all moral inhibitions. This gives the person a chance ultimately to make courageous decisions and undertake prudent actions based on *thoughts purposefully directed* towards the person who is the cause of the suffering.

It will be important to support Mr H carefully in both the distracting and directed movements of thought. He needs to avoid a flare-up of resentment against Susanne, because he cannot release himself from her in a state of resentment, and at the same time he needs to secure an inner distance from her, which will allow him to move on with hope.

Schönfeld: How is Mr H to get back on his feet? The first thing he must do is to address something that he has neglected for three years, namely the management of his own life. A life with well-cultivated friendships and self-chosen tasks. One goal is for him to go to bed in the evening able to confirm that his day was spent in a meaningful way. Another goal is to get up in the morning with the intention of tackling whatever may await him in the dawning day. He soon comes up with acquaintances from the past that he could contact again. It is possible that they are annoyed that he hasn't made contact for so long. But he could try to get in touch with them again.

I talk to him about another idea. Only those who can live a stable life on their own are capable of living stably with another person. This surprises Mr H. He says that since he moved out of his parents' home after school and until he moved in with Susanne, he always lived with a partner. He never had an apartment of his own. He did not know how to live well alone. After a little thought, he agrees with me: it would represent progress if he could live on his own and be content...but he doesn't have the self-confidence for this. He rejects the idea.

In our next session, he reports that he phoned two former friends. They, did not, however, seem to want to have anything to do with him. They were happy to hear from him, but no meeting was suggested. Before he sinks into further misery (everyone else is the problem!) I suggest that he can be the one to take the initiative and propose a meeting. He must accept the risk that the suggestion will be rejected. He should look beyond his own grief and begin to take an interest in other people, to ask how they are, to empathise with their situation. Also, he should be communicating with all sorts of people who have nothing to do with Susanne; the world is larger than his fixation on her suggests.

I offer him the metaphor of two living rooms. His last three years are represented by *one* of these rooms. How was this room furnished? Susanne's presence was all it could hold. Then there was his dog and the walks he took with it. There was also his job and Susanne's family. That was it. He is currently situated in the most difficult place: the threshold between this room, which he must leave, and a *second* room, which he must now enter, for better or worse. He avoids entering it, because this new living room is almost completely empty, not yet furnished so that it feels comfortable. What should he put in there? Mr H has no idea. I gently remind him that the gym is already in it, as well as the temporary accommodation with his parents. Of course, this is not enough. He is frightened by the emptiness. However, this emptiness also means the freedom to design his future room himself according to his own taste and style. He doesn't have to adopt any traditional models, he doesn't have to follow in anyone else's footsteps, he has a wonderful thing: freedom of choice!

Lukas: A standard method of logotherapy is to point out the existence of spiritual freedom. In hardened areas it may be necessary to open this freedom up backwards before it can be opened forwards. The metaphor of the two rooms is a good example. The room representing Mr H's recent past is full of open spaces that he did not use to good effect. He *had* the freedom to maintain a happy relationship with his parents. He *had* the freedom to integrate friendships into his conjugal life. He *had* the freedom to talk to Susanne about whether she was happy with their relationship. When it became clear that this was not the case, he *had* the freedom to ask her for time to find a small apartment for himself before moving out. In addition, he *had* the freedom to look for a suitable alternative home for his dog, if he could not keep it himself. In the course of the therapy, it will become clear that there were many other missed opportunities for making meaningful use of the space of freedom that existed for him in his old life.

From many years of experience, I can say that this insight can shake up a patient like Mr H in such a healing way that the freedom of the present is suddenly perceived in a rush of clarity. If this happens, he will immediately understand what the new room offers him: the opportunity to make considered and appropriate use of the freedom he has *now*. *Now* he has the freedom to thank his parents, to make friends, to forgive Susanne, to ask her where the dog is now, to look for a place to stay and to fulfil his duty to his patient employer by providing attentive customer service. To be confronted with one's space of freedom is "wonderful and terrible at the same time," as Frankl put it – terrible because it comes with a sudden recognition of great responsibility, but wonderful because one can put one's hand to the wheel and take part in steering the world.

Schönfeld: The next time Mr H came back, nothing had improved. He had not pursued the perspective of a way forward, he had still been unsuccessful in making any contacts, and he still cries all the time. He talks only about Susanne and describes her as an almost transcendent creature. I allow him one more "directed thought" before we return to distracting his thoughts away from Susanne. This directed thought should sharpen the realism of his vision.

When they first met, Susanne already had a boyfriend, whom she immediately abandoned for him. She had just completed her training as a sales assistant in a clothing store. For her 20th birthday, Susanne was given a traditional-style apartment in the city centre by her wealthy parents. The apartment needed a lot of renovation and had no furniture. Mr H paid for this renovation and furnishing on credit. He would give her anything...

"Anything"? Is that smart? Is that responsible? He would do "anything" for her – even if it made no sense? Would he murder, steal, commit acts of terrorism for her? Is this really love, a willingness to actually do "anything" for another human being? Or is that just infantile dependence? *Love does what is meaningful for a person.* It does what is good for *everyone* involved. It does what makes shared joys possible. "Anything", by contrast, includes anything destructive. I ask Mr H again what he means when he says he had been willing to do "anything" for his Susanne. We write down a long list of things that amount to spending a large sum of money. He looks at this list in silence for a while and shakes his head at himself. And *why* did he want to do "anything" for her? To avoid losing her? Well, in *that* case he has certainly miscalculated!

Fortunately, within this vortex of "anything", we discover that there was at least one of Susanne's wishes that he (meaningfully) resisted. She often said that she wanted to have a child with him. He had hesitated. After spending so much on the apartment, he had no financial resources left to spend on a child. This indicated a laudable sense of responsibility. So he *can* make responsible choices about how to use his space of freedom, even in the face of external pressure, and he will need this skill in the future. I don't want to tarnish his idealised image of Susanne, but his apparently boundless naivety clearly enabled her to exploit him. One person's weakness played into the other's, as is so often the case. Even now, Mr H says that Susanne can keep all the things in the apartment that he paid for. After all, he cannot fit them into the tiny room in which he is currently staying. Yes, and what about later on? What about some fair financial compensation?

He shakes his head. He would be at her feet again the moment she summoned him. I ask him about his "trust" in her. Perhaps he would succumb to her charms again, but would he ever really trust her again? He thinks about this and answers confidently: No! He would always expect to be shown the door at any moment. He could hardly just continue the relationship as if nothing had happened. His trust in her would have vanished! He would have to have good reasons to trust her again, and this is not the case at the moment. This visibly shakes him. Love cannot prosper without mutual trust. And he knows that.

Lukas: Mr H's assessment of Susanne as a "transcendent creature" is typical of a so-called pyramidal value system (Stanislav Kratochvil) in which there is a highest value sitting at the top of a pyramid of values. This highest, overvalued value is essentially worshipped, while all other values (Mr H's dog, his work, his family) are dismissed as secondary. Pyramidal value systems lead to reactive depression – at precisely the moment when the top of the pyramid breaks off. If the highest value is lost, the secondary values are too weak to support the person through the pain of this loss; thus the collapse into a "bottomless pit". Here we find the answer to the question we asked earlier: What were the elements of this crisis that caused Mr H to slip from natural grief into reactive depression? Immaturity, lack of attention to his space of freedom, infantile dependence and a pyramidal value system have combined to multiply his misfortune. Only a corrective rebalancing of his values in the direction of a parallel value system, in which many components of life are of equal value, can provide a sustainable platform for recovery. Therefore, the value "Susanne" must be progressively lowered, as the values of other components of his life are successively raised.

Schönfeld: During our next consultation, Mr H reports that he has removed Susanne's phone number and e-mail address from his phone. He stopped taking the antidepressants on his own initiative, without asking his doctor. He has recycled all the clothes Susanne ever gave him. He deleted all photos of her, and threw all gifts from her away. After that, he slept well for the first time in weeks. His doctor – who understandably did not like that he had abruptly stopped taking the antidepressents (they should be phased out slowly, because abrupt withdrawal is difficult for the body) – has signed him off sick for one last period; after that he wants to resume work. These were not balanced reactions, but they did at least represent a turning away from the era of his dependence through independent steps taken in freedom. There is only a thin whiff of resentment; we have avoided an escalation to full-scale anger.

In the following weeks, we worked on taking two further steps. For one thing, Mr H is able to look back without bitterness on the three happy years with Susanne. The relationship between the two young people was not exemplary, but he loved her intensely, and he should be able to remember this period more positively than mournfully. I take some time to question and expand a little on his concept of love. We ask: What should a successful relationship look like? After all, he had already experienced and ended many relationships with women before he met Susanne and she finally threw him out.

So what can bring permanence and sustainability in our transitory and rapidly changing times? We consider possible answers.

Our second major theme is the furnishing of his new living room, which continues to be a laborious undertaking. Finally he succeeds in reviving an old contact with one of his cousins. His cousin is married and has children. My patient likes to visit him. The cramped living situation with his parents continues to be unsatisfactory. But he has re-established a personal relationship with them. As soon as his debts are paid, which will take a few more months, he is determined to find his own apartment. He dreams about moving to the country, because he longs to have a dog again, and he would get more exercise there than in the city. In the meantime, he is looking into dog breeds and researching breeders on the internet, which a clear indication that his wound is slowly healing.

Lukas: When a person is in the middle of a painful situation, it may seem completely devoid of meaning, as if higher powers were playing cruel games. Even spiritually well-anchored persons can sometimes be very angry with their God and his acts when disasters happen. However, as time passes, this opinion can change drastically. Surprisingly often, decades later, sufferers say that in retrospect they *can* see a meaning in their past suffering, or can recognise that some good and valuable things came out of their terrible experience. Some say, "I've grown enormously from that experience." Others say, "It threw me off track and set me on an unexpected path that I would never have taken otherwise, but which makes me feel happy and fortunate now." Or, they say, "It has given me an acute understanding and sympathy for other people in similar situations."

I am sure that Mr H will experience the same thing. There will come a day in his future life when he will be glad of what he now regrets. He will humbly understand what he needed to learn through this suffering, and he will thankfully appreciate the magic that lay in this new beginning.

Schönfeld: Mr H has returned to work. He finds it difficult, but the hours in which he manages to focus on his insurance customers help him and steady him. They provide a respite from the dark memories with which he is still wrestling.

It took him about six months in total to regain some stability and overcome his depression. His new "living room" is gradually becoming comfortable. It includes evenings in the gym. Unfortunately, he still has limited social contact, but he has various plans to address this. Perhaps he will spend a summer holiday with an old school friend who has moved to Portugal. He could find out more about his family. He would try to learn a few phrases in Portuguese. Why not? He is also considering a professional change of direction. His professional experience would get him job and promotion opportunities at several major insurance agencies. Continuing education is at the top of his list of future projects.

His plans are still vague, but they are gradually taking shape. His sphere of interest has markedly increased, and this is unmistakable evidence that his psychic wounds are healing.

Dealing with Anxiety

Lukas: The theologian Eugen Bieser once described fear as the fundamental feeling of our time. Of course, "our time" is a broad term. Also, the "fundamental feelings" of the many different peoples of our world are by no means all the same. Nevertheless, there is a grain of truth in Bieser's claim. Average anxiety levels have actually increased. There have not been many statistical studies of anxiety in poverty-stricken countries and deprived areas. However, in places where there is no guarantee of day to day survival, it would be understandable for basic fears to control behaviour. The anxiety of the relatively well-off inhabitants of wealthy areas, in contrast, is more surprising. This can be seen not only in lively internet discussions on the subject, but also in scientific studies that show a worrying increase in anxiety disorders. We can only conclude that prosperity does not really relieve anxiety. This can be understood insofar as wealth always raises the anxious question of what would happen if it were to be lost. The more dependent humanity becomes on anything, be it possessions, databases, energy suppliers, computer processors, or anything else, the more it must worry that the failure of these economic and technological aids could provide a setback. And as the world's current political, climatic and ecological structures hardly seem stable, we can begin to understand how an anxious pessimism weighs on the minds of many and robs the privileged classes of their *joie de vivre*.

Now only privileged people can afford psychotherapeutic help. It is a genuine luxury to be able to entrust your worries and fears to a competent counsellor, and it is a great happiness if this counsellor finds the right words to reduce the weight of these psychic burdens. The "right words" that fit the situation often include a reminder reminiscent of the biblical commandment: "You are free to eat from any tree in the garden; but you must not eat from the tree of the knowledge of good and evil..." This is it: "You may hope for everything, but *you must not expect anything*!" To elaborate: "You must not expect anything pleasant (in a complaining way) because it sets you up for bitter disappointments, and you must not expect anything unpleasant (as a prophecy) because it fuels your fears." Viktor E. Frankl, the great doctor of the soul, cleverly expressed this appeal through a change of perspective, establishing the maxim: "What matters is never what you expect from life, but only what life expects from you!"

While expectation makes people passive and puts them at the mercy of circumstances beyond their control, the consciousness that something important and meaningful is expected *from them* makes

70

them active, ready and courageous. The question is not what other people would expect and want from you, but – as Frankl has clearly emphasised – what is expected from you "on behalf of life". One could also say: for the sake of a successful outcome for all, for living together in peace, for dignity and decency, ethos and *logos*. Focussing on what could be the best possible thing that is called for and required in the particular current situation does not eliminate all fears, but it relegates them to the background of thought, where they have less influence. Come what may, there will always be something that life is asking of you, and it will always be "good" to comply with this request. No matter how external circumstances change, you will always possess the opportunity to do so. If there is any consolation in troubled times, it is this.

Using a case study from her extensive psychotherapeutic practice, my colleague outlines how Frankl's maxim can be usefully applied to a case of confusion.

Schönfeld: Mrs I is 42 years old. There is sometimes tension in her relationship with her husband, but she sticks to it: she has married "the love of her life". Her two children are doing well in school. The family is intact. Both parents have successful careers and enjoy their work. They have built a small house in the country and they have every reason to be happy and content.

Mrs I has been suffering from severe back pain for some time. She has been receiving specialist treatment for almost three years, but so far this has brought her little relief. In the end, her orthopaedist suggested that perhaps the cause of her problems was psychic, and he recommended psychotherapeutic treatment. This is why she has come to me. She immediately explains that, in her opinion, some things are not quite as they should be with her work and family.

Our first topic of conversation is her marriage. Mrs I loves her husband. Nothing much has changed since she met him for the first time twenty years ago and immediately fell in love with him. Unfortunately, over the years, many of their interactions have become empty rituals. Their feelings for one another have partly cooled. She and her husband talk a lot about their relationship and how they think it should be different; they talk about what is wrong and what they expect from each other. But they just go round in circles and end up more unhappy than ever after a few hours. Mrs I concludes her lament: *if* her husband would ask more often about her work, *if* he would be a little more passionate, *if* he would pay more attention to their difficult adolescent son...then everything would be fine.

I ask Mrs I to think about this: in our time it is very common to have expectations of others – and to expect others to fulfil them. But a closer look reveals that our expectations quickly push other people into a corner. We immediately understand this if we experience it ourselves. When someone insistently and strongly expects something specific from us, we immediately put out our "inner spikes". For example, we would have happily baked a birthday cake if it had not been demanded from us. Or, we would have liked to have offered an invitation, if it had not been for the reproach: "Why can't you invite us over for once!" Our desire to be generous suddenly vanishes. Gifts that are demanded can no longer be gifts; against a horizon of expectations they become a compulsory tax, in which even the demander can no longer really take pleasure, because the gifts are given against the giver's will. In a relationship, expectations paralyse independent initiative. They put a cloud of pressure over everything that could have come from the heart. In conclusion, I suspect that such things have crept into many of the little nooks and crannies of Mr and Mrs I's relationship and dimmed their mutual love.

Mrs I confirms that this may well be so, and adds that her fruitless expectations probably also leave her physically cramped, which may affect her back. A change of attitude would be attractive to her. Free from all expectations and free to go through life on her own sovereign terms, independently of how her husband or her colleagues behave – she would like that! We conceive a program to "reduce all expectations to zero". Between now and our next session, she is willing to try the experiment of leaving all expectations of her husband aside and simply observing very carefully *how he is doing*, what would make *him* happy, what *he* does particularly well, and what they could enjoyably do together. Her partner should be relieved of the burden of responsibility for *her* well-being. In the future, she will manage this herself by practicing self-care. This will enable her to be more independent of whether someone else is noticing and taking into account what would please her.

Lukas: The American slogan "Expect nothing – appreciate everything" is a perfect summary of the psychotherapeutic intervention described above. It is a basic pedagogical rule never to tell a client or student what *not* to do, without also saying what should be done *instead*. The American slogan tells us not to expect, but instead to appreciate. It is characteristic of Frankl's teaching to direct attention to the outside world and its needs, and therefore away from one's own needs and the dogged habit of declaring that the outside world is responsible for meeting them. Mrs I is well advised to quash her expectations of her husband in favour of attention to his state, qualities and loveable nature. I am convinced that this will quickly have a good effect on their situation.

However, Mrs I will have to work hard at developing herself. Changes of habit are difficult and involve many relapses. Also, the phenomenon of collusion often takes root in relationships between two people. This term is borrowed from legal jargon, where it refers to deception and obfuscation. In psychological terminology, it refers to a process by which someone allows another person to support their (possibly idealised) self-image. The other person is "used" to shore up one's own self-image, which is an "obfuscation of the true motive". For example, in order to be able to sacrifice oneself (repeatedly), one requires a (continuously) needy person. In order to be able to wallow in suffering (continually), one requires a committed (and undaunted) helper. In order to be dominant, one needs a weak person who never grows out of this weakness. In all this, there is a more or less conscious calculation: the individual influences someone else in order to obtain a desired affirmation or "caress".

In therapy, it is necessary to lift these manipulations clearly into the consciousness and to undertake a ruthless enquiry into their meaningfulness. Manipulations may, for example, be described thus: "I stubbornly emphasise my mistakes in order to hear a clear confirmation from my partner that I am beyond fault or reproach." Or: "I pretend to be incompetent so that my boss takes difficult work away from me."Or: "I complain all the time to get tender words of comfort from my girlfriend." Or: "I live recklessly, so that my parents confirm again and again that they will rescue me from every scrape." *Is this meaningful?*

Logically, radical behavioural changes mean the end of any collusion that feeds on the absence of change in either person. By bravely renouncing the longed-for "caresses" and accepting a change in their self-image, individuals can liberate their "abused" partner from the compulsion to react in a certain way. Of course, the other party can also break the manipulation by reacting unexpectedly. If, for example, the boss gives the person who is feigning incompetence more difficult work for the sake of development, or if the parents tell their reckless son that he will have to solve his problems from now on, such collusions collapse.

Frankl's logotherapy is often referred to as a *discovering* therapy, in contrast to Sigmund Freud's *uncovering* therapy. It helps people to discover ways in which they can act meaningfully in the world, instead of always blindly reacting. In addition to being a *discovering* therapy, it is an *awakening* therapy, because it awakens an impulse for attitudinal and behavioural changes, which are needed to break away from established tracks and act independently and responsibly while forsaking desired reciprocal actions from others.

I do not know whether Mrs I "needed" a husband who did not meet her expectations in order to be able to shower him with accusations. Or whether Mr I "needed" a chronically frustrated wife in order to be able to ignore her constant demands in good conscience. It is unlikely, and we don't want to over-interpret anything. *If*, however, the two were entangled in such confused (unconscious?) manoeuvring, there could be no better emergency exit than the "prescription" administered by my colleague.

Schönfeld: Two weeks later, Mrs I reported that she had been struggling with the experiment, because it involved fighting against deeply entrenched patterns of behaviour. "But it feels right when it works," she tells me. At dinner, she listened more to her husband and asked him how things were going at work. She talked about their children without making any demands. Their conversations soon became more varied and interesting. Family life became easier, more cheerful and more pleasant. Mrs I wants to keep to this path. The austere and determined woman even feels some of her physical tension ebbing away as she loosens the reins on her strict way of life.

One habit has particularly changed. She admits that she often waited on her husband to provide an adequate demonstration of his love. Similarly, she waited to see whether her colleagues were sufficiently polite to her, whether her boss rewarded her achievements with appropriate recognition, and so on. She has now turned that around. She understands that no one can force love and praise from others. So she has withdrawn her energy from lurking in expectation and converted it into attentiveness. She has posed herself the following question: How can I encounter my husband, my children, and my colleagues in an appreciative and friendly way? Where can I offer a kind word, where can I lend a helping hand? Mrs I reports that this reversed perspective is very good for her. She is surprised how much her interactions with others – and thereby her own life – have relaxed.

Although so much has improved in her everyday life, which is now running smoothly, she now reports an issue that she has not yet mentioned. She finds it difficult to talk about. She has been suffering from panic attacks for more than a decade. These began when her mother was seriously ill at home for almost a whole year. The illness could have been fatal, but her mother eventually recovered. Mrs I had long since moved away from home; she had two small children, and was about to build a house with her husband. It was clear that she needed to look after her father. The problem was not that he needed a carer, explains Mrs I. He also had domestic help. What he could not deal with, however, was the mental suffering – it almost crushed him. At that time, as she spoke almost daily on the phone with him, he always poured out his heart about his great unhappiness, crying and complaining all the while.

This was when her panic attacks began. They came out of nowhere, with no immediate cause, and took her breath away. The only thing she could think of during an anxiety attack was that she might die from panic.

Lukas: It is not at all rare for patients to reveal their most pressing problems to a therapist only after a relationship of trust has been established. At first, they often test the waters with more superficial matters, to see if they can really dare to open themselves up to another person and divulge "secrets" of which they are perhaps ashamed. It is a bit surprising when Mrs I's anxiety neurosis comes to light during the course of her treatment. She is portrayed as a rather demanding, austere and determined woman, so one might expect her to evoke fear in others. However, one thing has pointed to hidden fears right from the beginning, namely the somatic effects of the psychic problems suspected by her orthopaedist. Strong fears tend to break through the outer boundary of the emotional realm and enter into the physical level of the body, where they weaken the immune system and cause all sorts of damage. Typical examples are vegetative psychosyndromes and anything that can be attributed to an overexcitation of the sympathetic nervous system, such as muscle tension (e.g. back pain), heart palpitations or an increased need for oxygen (e.g. breathing difficulties).

The worst thing is that the triggers of strong fears can disappear without the strong fears disappearing along with them. This means that, by appearing, triggers are responsible for initiating an undesirable development, but unfortunately, when they disappear, they do not end it. The classic example of this is a teenager who starts smoking as a result of peer pressure. He or she will probably continue to smoke even when this peer group has been forgotten.

For this reason, in the case of many exaggerated fears, addictions or bad habits, there is little point in searching for the original triggers. This knowledge does not impart freedom.

Mrs I already knows what triggered her panic attacks: her mother's serious illness and her father's exaggerated suffering. Well, maybe. Maybe not. Two things stand out in her story. On the one hand, her father's behaviour was clearly desperate. Of course the threat of losing of a spouse and the agony of having to watch this process are very difficult. However, Mrs I's father also put an enormous burden on his daughter. Perhaps he had a predisposition to anxiety disorder? This suggests that Mrs I's response could have a *hereditary* component. Or perhaps Mrs I's father is acting as a bad *role model* for her. The second possibility builds on the first. Did Mrs I have *feelings of guilt* for leaving her mentally overburdened father alone with his suffering? She had moved away from home and had started a family of her own, but her father was crying and complaining... "I'm not rushing to his aid," she might have thought. A predisposition and a bad role model – more than enough to result in panic.

Schönfeld: I ask her in detail her about her panic attacks. Nothing concrete comes out of this conversation, however. The only thing that can be discerned in Mrs I's panic attacks is a vague fear of her own death.

There were some bad periods in her life when these panic attacks occurred up to ten times a day, but there were also weeklong periods free from panic. She cannot explain when and why her attacks were more or less frequent. The only thing she has noticed is that she never has a panic attack when she is with other people (when she is distracted from herself). During working hours, an attack may occur when she goes to the toilet – that is, when she is alone for a few minutes. Sometimes she wakes up at night with her barometer of emotions fluctuating wildly. This has caused her to develop a strong *fear of fear*. "I hope I won't have a panic attack today," is the first thing she thinks when she leaves home early in the morning. She tries to be alone as little as possible; this (apparently) protects her.

We talk for a while about the inevitability of death, towards which all biological life is heading. Of course it is sad that she will die one day, but is it a reason to panic now? We differentiate between "good" fears that help to preserve our lives – for example, when we are afraid to cross a road in the midst of heavy traffic. "Good" fears tend to push away the inevitability of death, because they keep in check our willingness to take risks. Thus, we should keep our "good" fears. Is her panic a "good" fear? No, it doesn't help her, it doesn't protect her from anything – on the contrary, it has a very negative effect on her life. *Therefore, the panic should be rejected.*

The origin of "bad" fears, as opposed to "good" fears, is only of limited interest. One can speculate about it, but even if one knows exactly where they come from, it does not answer the question of how to get rid of them. Mrs I's panic attacks manifested themselves for the first time in the context of severe psychological stress, but thousands of people are exposed to severe psychological stress without developing panic attacks as a result. One has to understand that inappropriate, "bad" fears can barge into one's life out of nowhere, even in the absence of difficulties.

The question of how to evict these fears from everyday life is much more important than speculating about their origins. Viktor E. Frankl created a highly effective tool for this purpose, which is his method of paradoxical intention. This method is based on two simple facts.

1. No one can fear and wish for and the same thing at the same time – fear and desire are mutually exclusive. One cannot, for example, be afraid that the police will ring the doorbell, and at the same time fervently wish for them to do so. Desire and fear block one another.

2. Another two things that are mutually exclusive are fear and humour. No one can laugh out loud with pleasure and shudder in fear at the same time. Again, these two things block one another.

The method of paradoxical intention makes use of these two facts by encouraging the patient to provoke and ridicule one's own unnecessary fear of panic and all of its threatening gestures. The fear is then *blocked in two ways*: by both the (paradoxical) desire and the (paradoxical) humour. This double blockade cannot be broken even by deeply-rooted inherited or acquired sensitivities, which simply melt away.

I tell Mrs I about a little trick that will help us with this melting-away project. It is easier to face the raging fear bravely and mess around with it if we give it as funny a name as possible. I try out some possibilities that harmonise with Mrs I's own fantasies, until we find a suitable expression. From now on, the dreaded panic attack is to be called "the grasshopper", because it tries to *scare* her by jumping out at her suddenly, because it has a startling appearance, and reminds her a bit of *grasshoppers* that ravage everything in sight in large swarms. We flesh out her imaginative picture: the grasshopper is very ugly, says Mrs I, it is black and has a large number of horrible legs.

Lukas: A biblical scholar once told me that in the Bible the command "do not be afraid" occurs exactly 364 times, almost one time for each day of the year. Whether or not this is a coincidence, it shows that people have struggled with fear since the beginning of time.

As my colleague correctly explained to her patient, fear normally has a protective *function*. None of our songbirds would survive if they settled on people's shoulders and windowsills without fear. They would be plucked, roasted, fried, caged or abused as children's toys... Unfortunately, however, biologically meaningful fears can begin to reproduce in humans like cancer cells. Technically, one speaks of irrational fears, which are no longer appropriate to the current situation. If the growth of these fears is not stopped, they can become dangerous and even form something analogous to metastases. At first, a person is afraid of driving a car, then afraid of getting on buses and trains, then afraid of entering offices, restaurants, etc. until in the end, the sheer "fear of fear" becomes a life-dominating tyrant.

The danger of allowing irrational fears to proliferate is threefold:

1. They increasingly inhibit the individual in all activities. Some of the person's thoughts are constantly being led away from the things and tasks that he or she actually wishes to pursue. The person's head becomes full of all the horrible things that can and will happen. Everything else becomes secondary, and the person becomes distracted and fidgety. Even at night, there is little rest.

2. Irrational fears magically attract the very thing that is feared. It is an irony of fate that a fearful person often experiences the very calamity that he or she wants to avoid at any cost. For example, if a man is afraid of being cheated on by his partner, he might exasperate her with his jealousy until she leaves him. People who are afraid of doing badly in a job interview may come across so insecurely that they are rejected.

3. Strong existential fears lead one away from meaning. Much of the evil, hatred, social coldness, and destructive behaviour in the world is initiated by fear. This can be seen most clearly in the rise of xenophobia, but even in less blatant derailments we see how defensive movements set in motion by massive fears often affect innocent people and spread suffering.

For Mrs I, so far only the first point is relevant, which is a good reason to resist fear from the outset. Hints of the third point might be seen in her insistent need for proofs of love from her husband or recognition from her boss. Fear whispers in her ear, "Are you loved at all? Are you appreciated? Are you 'somebody' or 'nobody'"? Anyone who takes such a whisper seriously looks for reassurance.

One of Frankl's most ingenious ideas was to tap into the human capacity for self-distancing in order to decouple anxiety sufferers from the spectres evoked by their fears; to distance the sufferer from the fear. People who feel inseparably united with their fears, indeed, almost obsessed with them, are completely at their mercy. However, as soon as they move away from their fears in spirit and place themselves at a fruitful distance from them, they can defeat them, direct them, mock them, summon them, toss them away, trample them underfoot, humiliate them – in short, they can do anything that one might do to an adversary, in particular, a defeated adversary. The irrational fear shrinks into a dwarf-size that the person can deal with.

Schönfeld: From now on, Mrs I becomes the one who torments *"the grasshopper"*, and she learns to ridicule it cheerfully. I practice with her, instructing her to give orders to the imaginary representative of her fear. We tell the grasshopper to squat under a chair in the corner and ridicule it because it has already weakened so much. At her prime, she induced panic in Mrs I almost ten times a day, and now she is hard pressed to bring about five attacks. This is inferior work! What is the point of a grasshopper that has lost its ability to startle? It must do better, otherwise it will be shown the door! We formulate a daily plan to increase its efficiency. What does Mrs I plan to do after her session with me? She will do some shopping in a supermarket twenty minutes from here, and then she has a ten mile drive to get home. This is the plan we make for the grasshopper. It should provide a first-class panic attack with all the trimmings right at the entrance to the shopping centre. Exactly there, not ten feet before or after. We require careful work! And that's just a warm up. On the ten mile journey home, the grasshopper should deliver a nice little panic attack every three miles, a sequence of three attacks. That will be enough for today, but tomorrow at breakfast it will be given new instructions.

Mrs I does not know what to do with this (paradoxical) banter, which is so contrary to her intentions, but she cannot resist a smile. I "put her in command" over the grasshopper. She should grab it by the collar and hang it out of the car window if it does not behave itself. If the grasshopper presents too gloomy an appearance, its black legs can be painted in bright colours. Dwarf sized creatures should also keep up with fashion. The grasshopper must follow Mrs I everywhere, staying a submissive two feet behind her. Only the marriage bed is off limits; only Mrs I's husband is allowed there. The bed is a grasshopper-free zone. The many-legged beast must wait outside the door at night.

Mrs I cannot stop smiling in amazement. She looks a little expectant and suspicious, but she is willing to play along with the grasshopper story. She masters the art of turning the tables and play-fully wishing for what she fears. *She* is now the one in charge; she can defy her fear and order it about, and she should do this with a large dose of humour. If she smiles even a little, she has already won – monsters like her grasshopper cannot withstand this at all; they shrivel up at once.

Mrs I hesitates a little, then heroically "collects" her grasshopper from under the chair and orders it into the back seat of her car. "If you're not well-behaved and obedient, I'll stuff you in the exhaust pipe," she mutters and drives off.

Lukas: I know that, like Mrs I, the readers of this story may feel that this humorous approach to therapy is not a good idea. At first, it is hard to believe that the method of paradoxical intention is useful and will lead to positive results. I can assure you, however, that it will. There is much more to a human being than a palette of feelings. In particular, feelings which do not arise from the values of the spirit (as love does in its most beautiful form), but from the influence of psychic drives and conditioning, can only claim leadership if this claim is uncontested. Some feelings simply have to be contradicted, because they are inappropriate. They do not contribute to making life more agreeable, which is their purpose. If someone feels thirsty, for example, then this indicates a genuine need for hydration. The feel-ing of thirst may cause one to drink. If an alcoholic thirsts for alco-hol, however, then this is merely a sign of addiction. The feeling suggests that it would be agreeable to drink more alcohol, *but this is not the case*. The feeling must therefore not be allowed to lead to alcohol consumption, and this means that it needs to be resisted.

It is the same with feelings of fear. There are realistic, appropriate feelings of uneasiness that warn of real threats, and against which we can have no objection. However, there are also unnecessary feelings of panic, which are not appropriate. One must not give into them or consider their false warnings to be valid. The drama staged with the help of paradoxical intention quickly reveals their emptiness: if one goes forth to meet the threatened outcomes courageously with mocking desire, nothing bad happens. The only result is the relief of a enslaved person who has cowered for far too long under a non-existent sword of Damocles – which then somehow falls, enticed by fear alone (see point 2 above).

Schönfeld: When Mrs I comes back two weeks later, the first thing I ask is whether she has brought along her grasshopper. I'm very curious to find out: has she found the courage and humour to reduce the panic attacks that have plagued her for years, perhaps even to leave them behind? Mrs I replies, laughing, that she does not know what is happening. She thinks she must have accidentally left the grasshopper with me under the chair in the corner and it did not get into her car at all, as she ordered. Mrs I has not suffered *a single panic attack* since our last session; she has experienced no fear of death and she has slept soundly every night – there has been no sign of the grasshopper at all! She does not understand, and her husband is just as surprised. She can't imagine that a single therapeutic conversation would have achieved all of this, but of course she is very relieved that her panic attacks have vanished. She admits that two weeks ago she still had doubts about my proposal. Nevertheless, she had decided to try it. She had conducted comical conversations with the personification of her fear, teasing the grasshopper mercilessly – and the grasshopper had actually vanished. "What do I have to lose," Mrs I had thought, and she had played along with the joke.

I am thrilled. I am used to Frankl's therapy methods working efficiently, but often patients need repeated instructions and a lot of training, and some need a lot of patience, practice and encouragement. Mrs I is an amazing exception. However, I must honestly tell her that her fears may spring up at some point again, whether tomorrow, or in twenty years. She carries this possibility inside herself. Now, however, she also knows how to get rid of such fears. If they ever rise up again to taunt her, she can chase them away in no time. What she has learned in the past weeks, equips her permanently to put an end to all the grasshopper's descendants, using humour and paradox. We repeat the basic exercise again: 1. Notice when fears become exaggerated. 2. Distance yourself from them and give them a ridiculous name. 3. Never again retreat from such fears with cowardice. 4. Rather, smile, drag them out of their hiding place, and converse with them. 5. Ask them what exactly they want to scare you with. 6. Whatever the answer may be, accept it happily and cheerfully. ("You are threatening me with immediate death? Fine, today I will die three times in a row. You go first, then me, then you again, then me, and so on. So go on then, I will follow you right away!") 7. *Do not take seriously what does not deserve to be taken seriously.* Real life is difficult enough without adding irrational problems to it. Serenity and cheerfulness quickly put an end to these.

I am very proud of Mrs I. Some women have jewellery and furs, but she has something more precious. She has the experience that she "doesn't have to put up with everything that comes out of her (and her weaknesses)". Nothing is so uplifting as a victory over oneself.

A year later, I receive a happy email from her in which she thanks me exuberantly: a year has passed, and the effect has continued. The grasshopper has shown itself no more! Mrs I is happy and relieved.

I am also relieved – but I am not really surprised. I know that logotherapeutic methods work in the long term. Once patients have learned how to "pull themselves out of the swamp by their hair," they no longer need a therapist.

Dealing with Compulsive Thoughts

Lukas: As living creatures, we are subject to a number of constraints. To survive, we need to eat and drink. We need to breathe. We need to avoid excessively hot or cold temperatures. The list is long... and death always threatens. Animals and plants are no different: "To be or not to be?" is the lifelong question, until finally non-being prevails.

For us humans, however, there exists another dimension: *the spiritual dimension*, as Viktor E. Frankl called it in accordance with age-old traditional thought. It could also be called the dimension of spiritual freedom, because it opens a window onto freedom between the natural constraints which restrict us. There we have the space to make our own spiritually free decisions, to set ourselves personal goals, to perform the actions of our choice, to adopt our own opinions, to search for meaning, to make value judgements and to believe in something or in someone out of choice. In this window, we are *more* than descendants of plants and animals; there, we are children with a spiritual home.

Consequently, we always protest with the greatest violence if we experience constraints in the "window". At an early age, as our spirit slowly awakens, we resist our parents' attempts to control us. Later, we resent superiors and authorities if they impose on us too much. Every state loses the loyalty of its citizens if it puts them in a dictatorial straitjacket. Coercion has never been a suitable means to create or maintain social peace. It frustrates the born rights of the human spirit and incites it to rebellion.

A particularly tragic and unpleasant form of compulsion is *self-compulsion*. Because the human being mysteriously unites nature and spirit, it is possible for biological or psychological addictions to enter the window and begin to obstruct it. Illnesses often narrow the human sphere of action, but some illnesses consist of nothing more than a frontal attack on the freedom of the spirit. These include *addictions* and *obsessive-compulsive disorders*. By means of neural processes and emotional "blackmail" they gain access to the human will and gradually break it. What is left is often a miserable human wreck, hardly capable of rebellion. The human spirit resigns. And this gives non-being the upper hand over being...

In contrast to dementia, which also limits spiritual freedom, addictions and obsessive-compulsive disorders are treatable and eliminable. But it is not easy! Not easy for the therapist, and certainly not for the sufferer. Although it takes no time to slip into an addiction, it takes an almost endless amount of "defiance of the spirit" (Frankl) – as well as patience and perseverance – to climb out of it again. Sufferers of obsessive-compulsive disorders are no better off. Often, the burden of their hereditary predisposition has meant that the years since their adolescence have been a slippery slope, in which their thoughts have always been plagued by the same banalities, they have buckled under the weight of abstruse fears, and they have not learned or even tried to defend themselves against their own compulsive thoughts. The spiritual "window" bangs open and shut in the storm of desperate feelings.

Schönfeld: In psychotherapeutic practice, obsessive-compulsive disorders are often amongst the most difficult and arduous challenges. I can testify to that. But the opposite can also be true. With the help of Frankl's ingenious methods, it is sometimes possible to release sufferers from their torments through a single logotherapeutic intervention. I recently had this experience twice in a row and would like to describe how it happened.

Report 1:
A 23 year-old woman, Ms J, comes to me with teary eyes and tells me, full of despair, that she is "afraid of everything". She was afraid even as a little girl. For example, if she woke up at night, she was

afraid. In this case, she was allowed to crawl into her parents' bed, which soothed her. She still worries a lot, only now there is no longer a protected cave to snuggle in. For example, what would happen if she became dizzy while driving? Sometimes she thinks so hard about this frightening possibility that she actually does get slightly dizzy.

A few weeks ago, she had a bad experience. She was out partying with a group of friends when one of them pulled a joint out of his pocket and offered it around. Not everyone took it, but she took three drags, because she had been told that it made one completely relaxed and carefree. She wanted to feel this relaxation once. Under the influence of the drug, the others only became giggly and silly, but she had horrific visions as though she was in a horror film. Since then, she has been afraid that the horror film might recur.

She reports that two weeks ago, her closest friend died in a tragic motorcycle accident. Ms J had known her since kindergarten. The two had pursued the same career, but in different cities. For this reason, they talked to one another almost every day. Listening to this, I think that the young woman's greatest sorrow should be the sudden death of her friend. She cries when she talks about it, so I suggest that we talk about this severe shock first. But she dismisses the idea. No, her *biggest problem* is that she can't stop thinking about the joint. Is it because she took those three drags that she can no longer control her thoughts? Never again in her life will she touch drugs again... I ask about the horrible thoughts with which she plagues herself. "I thought for the first time that I could do something terrible to someone. Since then, this thought has haunted me; I can't get it out of my mind." At the same time, she swears that she never wants to do harm to anyone, not even an animal. She wouldn't even step on a beetle. Nevertheless, the thought goes round and round in her head: "You might do it *anyway!*" like a carousel that can't be stopped.

Lukas: One sign of all anxiety and obsessive-compulsive disorders is the *disproportionality* of the thoughts that preoccupy the sufferer.

They are simply out of proportion. Even a layman quickly notices the conspicuous excesses of these symptoms: too much brooding, too much fear, too much caution, too much attention, etc. What is missing is not so obvious, but it is also important. In the case my colleague described above, it is obvious enough. Ms J grieves far too little about the loss of her closest friend. And she has nothing to say about her interests, her career, or the social group to which she belongs.

It is obvious why these psychic disorders (which used to be called neuroses) flare up in phases of ease and tend to die away in times of disaster. If you lose your home to an earthquake or a flood, or if you have to pull yourself and your family through a life of bitter poverty, then there is little energy left to brood on or anticipate bad experiences. One has no leisure for excessive anxiety. Viktor E. Frankl expressed this in the following parable:

"...it is a matter of experience that situations of external distress and crisis are generally accompanied by a decrease in the incidence of neurotic illness, and even in the life of an individual person it is often the case that a strain in the form of a demand placed on the individual has a psychologically healthy effect. I always compare this with the fact that a dilapidated building can be supported and strengthened by a heavy load."[6]

Now the premature death of her friend had placed a burden on Ms J, but this did not take the form of a demand on her. If she had been required to arrange her friend's burial, manage her legacy and sell her apartment, the experience with the joint would probably have been forgotten. However, a therapist cannot "prescribe" demands of this kind; they only help if they arise from genuine necessities. There is a logotherapeutic method called dereflection, by which a patient's circling thoughts are interrupted by removing the centre around which

---

[6] Viktor E. Frankl, Theorie und Therapie der Neurosen, UTB Ernst Reinhardt, Munich, 2007, p. 144.

they circle. Unfortunately, this method is not enough to arrest strong fears. For this, there is only one efficient and immediately effective method (which we have already learned), the method of paradoxical intention. No doubt my colleague will draw on it right away.

However, once the strong fears have been banished, the best thing for the recovering patient is a large dose of dereflection. Their "dilapidated building" should be supported with many colourful projects and meaningful demands, so that the predisposition to neurosis has no opportunity to creep back in through the back door. Anne Fleck, a recovered sufferer, wrote this beautiful sentence: "The only way to know you are a winner in life is to forget yourself in devotion to others."[7] I can only applaud this.

Schönfeld: I inform Ms J that it she is experiencing not an effect of the drug, but compulsive thoughts. Compulsive thoughts thrive on our desire to push them away. But the more pressure you exert on them, the stronger their counter-pressure becomes – just like in physics: pressure creates counter-pressure. And also like in physics: if you fight, your opponent fights back. Ms J explains, "I only do this because I am so afraid of it... because it is so terrible!"

It is clear that Ms J wants to get rid of her compulsive thoughts, but let's think about the logic of this situation. If a desire to push them away exacerbates them, what would diminish them? "Not pushing them away?" asks Ms J timidly. "Exactly," I answer, "and you can go further and turn everything completely around: you even have to want them! In with the blackest of thoughts!"

Ms J protests: "I can't do it!" "Maybe you can," I encourage her. There is something else. Obsessions live on *two* things: the desire to push them away at all cost, and the huge fear that lies behind this. What is the logical response? The fear must also be defeated. Ms J. understands this. So, what can put a sudden end to fear? Funnily

---

[7] From the magazine Melchior No. 9/2018, Ch-6300 Zug / Switzerland.

enough – in the most literal sense – *a hearty laugh*! Fears cannot withstand being laughed at, it almost destroys them!

Now all we have to do is to wield these two weapons at once: a paradoxical desire for crude obsessions, and a healthy dose of humorous exaggeration. One might say: "Bring on your dark thoughts... it will put me in an excellent mood! Our Earth is overpopulated, so I will do something about it... with a kitchen knife today, a length of rope tomorrow, and the day after I'll use some rat poison... I'll kill anyone I can get my hands on!" Ms J laughs. This is good.

We have some fun imagining many possibilities. In our exaggeration, Ms J is supposed to "become a really bad girl". She laughs heartily. Deep down, she must have a cheerful nature, because these absurd exaggerations seem to stimulate the healthy parts of her. This ridiculousness will soon enable her to put her compulsive ideas to rest. Finally, she asks the question that all sufferers of compulsive disorders ask, as a result of their tendency to brood. Where does all this come from? Why do these awful imaginings afflict *me*?

The three drags on the joint cannot be held responsible for triggering them. However, we can point to Ms J's genes as a cause. Modern genetic research has shown that psychological dispositions are inherited, not just physical traits. We all carry certain predispositions to instability in us; risk factors that remain with us all our lives. Should we complain to our parents about this? They have only drawn from the gene pool of their ancestors – and Adam and Eve are too long gone to be accused. The most sensible thing to do is to strengthen and build up the protective factors that we also carry within us and find in our environment, and use them to contain these risk factors.

Lukas: What my colleague is talking about here used to be called an "anankastic character structure". Although this term is no longer used, there is no adequate alternative term. People with this predisposition are usually shining examples of reliability, love of order, cleanliness, and correctness. They want to do everything in an exemplary way, everything should provide 100% satisfaction, and if things get even a little tangled up, anankasts can easily go off the rails. Their spontaneity is impeded by their many scruples; but *when* they act, they do so deliberately and intentionally. A degree of perfectionism can be a professional advantage. Anankasts are punctual workers, cautious drivers, careful craftsmen, accurate dentists, they are agreeable and and pleasant people who can be trusted completely, and nothing is less likely for them than falling into criminal behaviour. If, however, these traits become excessive, cleanliness becomes compulsive washing, the love of order becomes an obsession with order, and in general, valid patterns of behaviour suddenly morph into a nightmare fear of perpetrating or being capable of perpetrating some horrible offence.

Absorbed in their fear of the imperfect, they try to rescue themselves by means of control mechanisms, which manifest themselves in the form of compulsive acts (and instead of saving them, these plunge them even deeper into the morass). They rub their fingers raw to avoid dirt, they check ten times before leaving home whether all appliances are switched off, or they ponder endlessly whether they have committed some misdemeanor or could so by mistake. They completely lack the internal security to do *nothing that they do not want to do*, which in technical jargon is referred to as an "inadequate sense of evidence" (Frankl). In the above example, Ms J is already dangerously close to this stage.

Because this type of character belongs to morally scrupulous people who "for God's sake" do not want to do anything wrong, there is no danger in instructing them to counter their most immoral nightmares with paradoxical declarations of intent. People like Ms J do not actually shoot or stab the people around them when they humorously decide to rid the world of superfluous inhabitants. All that happens is that their soul is freed from the superfluous ballast of their morbid thoughts. They leave no stoves or candles burning when they overcome themselves and leave home efficiently, protected by the paradoxical desire to leave a conflagration behind them.

Schönfeld: I say to Ms J, "No matter where your compulsive thoughts come from, whenever they appear, they are only useful for making fun of". Mrs Anxiety and Mr Compulsion are siblings who come along arm in arm. Ms J should take care to recognize the two in time. When does the miserable brooding begin? As soon as she spots them, she should greet them in a new way: "Hello, Mrs Anxiety, hello Mr Compulsion, nice to see you, let me give you a hug and a kiss!" These two can't stand this. They are used to being capitulated to with groans; they are not up to conducting a dialogue. We practice dialogues full of humour and exaggeration. Ms J transforms from being a slave of her feelings to being their mistress. *She* decides what the unfortunate siblings may and may not do. Our therapy session is hilarious, and Ms J is radiant. She likes this method.

I explain that it was very wise of her to take action in time when her compulsion was a baby just a few weeks old. This made it much easier to get rid of. She likes to laugh, and humour is her sharpest weapon. I also assure her that her *actual will* remains untouched by this parody. In reality, she does not want to harm anyone. *That* is the real her, *that* guides her through life. Crude obsessions like this always pounce on a person's highest values, because this is where they are the most aggravating. However, these compulsive thoughts are liars: they spin up fantasies that will never happen. And that is why one can make fun of them.

A week later, Ms J says that she is already much better. The compulsive thoughts have diminished and almost completely disappeared. I am pleased. How did she achieve this? "Well, just like you said. I didn't repress anything, I just exaggerated everything. If Mr Compulsion threatened that I would harm other people, then I answered him: "You are right, after lunch I will walk down the street with a serrated kitchen knife, knock on all the doors, and politely ask anyone who opens the door if I can cut their throats. Mr Compulsion had nothing to say to this. Once he turned up on the bus. I quickly dismissed him with the fantasy of mowing down all the passengers one by one."

What helped her to come up with these skillful responses? She stresses that it was important for her to realise that the fear-mongering is unreal, and does not correspond to her actual will. This emboldened her to meet it with a funny response. Praising her, I reiterate the main points of the method of paradoxical intention as a safeguard against relapses. One day, Mrs Anxiety and Mr Compulsion might once again rudely force their way into the midst of her thoughts – what should she do then? Of course, she will rub her hands and exclaim: "Hooray, it's time for a new joke!"

Ms J is no longer interested in this topic; she ticks it off her list even faster than I do. Now she is ready to reflect on other parts of her life and to find space to mourn the tragic loss of her friend.

Weeks later, she appears for a scheduled follow-up session. Her obsessive thoughts have completely vanished, and are literally *no longer worth talking about* for either of us.

Lukas: In the autumn of 2018, the German health insurance providers published statistics indicating that around a million children in Germany need therapy because of their psychic difficulties. At the same time, there was news that more than a million children had died of malnutrition in the civil war in Yemen. Looking at these two statistics side by side, one wonders if the German children might not be happy and grateful not to be hungry, but that is an ironic question. All children who lack proper nourishment for either body or spirit are poor.

Let us think about what children in industrialised nations who are in need of therapy are actually missing. According to the statistics, they suffer from a combination of exhaustion, anxiety, and depression. There may be various reasons for this. I would like to focus on two of them because they illustrate the polarity between freedom and compulsion.

Cause No. 1:
The children are vey good at using smartphones, but they have also become extremely dependent on them. Smartphones are "time-eaters". If children use them for three to five hours a day, other things fall by the wayside. These things include exercising, playing together (face to face), learning things by heart, and getting enough sleep. Not getting enough exercise or sleep is bad both for physical and mental fitness. Never playing together face to face is bad for social skills. And spending less time on learning leads to decreased performance at school, and this is bad for self-confidence. Children who are affected even slightly by "anankasm" – that is, the ones who are ambitious and hardworking – have considerable difficulty in meeting the demands of school as a result of their "time-eaters". These demands have not increased in recent decades, but the time available in each day to fulfil them has dropped alarmingly.

Cause No. 2:
To acquire social competence, children must rub up against one another and learn how to resolve conflict. This includes arguing with each other in the school playground or in the street. Social media, however, allows such conflicts to continue endlessly. They develop into hate speech and trolling on the internet. There is no longer a place of domestic intimacy into which children can escape, in which they are safe and where they can switch off. If parents have the time and mental energy to pick them up and comfort them, this is great, but parents are often subject to the same time pressure and exhaustion as their children. Who is surprised, then, that exhaustion, anxiety and depression are on the increase?

Humour is of limited help with this widespread problem. But there is another resource that enables us to withstand these attacks on human freedom, and that is *voluntary renunciation.* If one wanted to practice psychotherapy on a grand scale, it would be the industrialised nations (and not the starving ones) that would offer the best opportunities. It is not only children who would benefit from a reduction in their hours of electronic surfing. An army of addicts could recover merely by heroically renouncing the addictive substance. Sufferers of obsessive-compulsive disorders could largely recover by decisively renouncing all their striving for perfection. The worsening situations with microplastics in the food chain and pollution in the lungs of city dwellers would lose their apocalyptic character if there were a widespread willingness to enforce the renunciation of excessive waste, unnecessary driving, and so on, at a global level. I know that it is fantastical to speculate on these ifs, but I do not want to leave the issue of compulsion without having pointed out the importance of voluntary renunciation. The most terrible and unnecessary constraints are the ones that people have imposed on themselves. Spiritually, one can keep them in check, but only at the cost of renouncing something!

After this little digression, let us turn again to the individual stories and the therapeutic skill of my colleague.

Schönfeld: Ms J was lucky, because her obsessive thoughts had only recently broken into her (otherwise somewhat fearful) life. She immediately benefited from Frankl's helpful methods, and did not have to fight against deeply engrained compulsions, as many sufferers do. She also understood right away how paradoxical intention works. Torment became fun and playfulness; powerlessness became mastery.

Report 2:

About nine months before this, 64-year-old Mr K had come to me for therapy. He had played a lot of tennis in his youth, and had remained a keen tennis player all his life. At weekends he coached the youth team at the local tennis club.

Mr K came to me because of sleep problems When he lay in bed in the evening, he thought about tennis, and desperately tried to remember results from current grand slam tennis tournaments. A won his match 3:1 against B, C won 2:5 against D, etc. etc. Often, he also rehearsed in his mind the results of all the matches played by the youth team. If he couldn't remember the results, his sleep was "out the window," he said. He would fall asleep exhausted only towards morning and feel exhausted for all of the next day. Do I have a prescription for better sleep?

Sufferers of obsessive-compulsive disorders tend to hide their compulsions. They are ashamed of themselves, because they do not live in spiritual freedom, and they are even more ashamed of their fellow human beings, who never do more than shake their heads at their "nonsense". For this reason, sufferers of obsessive-compulsive disorders devise all sorts of artful tricks to shape their peculiar behaviour into more acceptable forms They may use words like burnout, bullying or depression to describe their misery – with Mr K it was his sleep problems I soon suspected that Mr K's disturbed nighttime hours were merely a *result* and not the *cause* of his suffering, but he insisted that he only wanted to talk about not being able to sleep.

To alleviate his fear of lying awake, the first thing I told him was that there is no need to worry too much about not sleeping a lot. The body is smart, and it gets the minimum amount of sleep it needs at a later time. It also falls into a deeper sleep in order to compensate for the reduced amount – quality replaces quantity. Mr K emitted an audible sigh of relief, and his panic subsided.

Second, I wanted to explore the root cause of his obsessive-compulsive disorder by testing his capacity for humour.

Reminiscences about tennis matches would be understandable, given his lifelong passion, I said, but having to remember the results of past matches every night is an ordeal and not a joy. How would it be to make this ordeal a game by cheerfully inventing fantasy tennis results like 43:27 or 105:0? Mr K was unimpressed: no, he was unable to change the numbers or have fun with them.

Third, I attempted a "dereflective detour" to stimulate his imagination. Could he play a memory match with himself at night? He would certainly have fond memories of places he had once been which had given him a feeling of security. Lying in a meadow watching butterflies fluttering on the flowers... sitting at the beach watching the crashing of the waves... feeling peace and inner calm... if he could revisit these places in his wakeful periods and imagine them in detail, he would soon be filled with the same peace he had before, and he would have a respite from the torment of tennis scores. Mr K was hesitant. His passion had always been for exciting matches rather than dull landscapes. The only thing that calms him is my assertion that his body will "somehow" get enough sleep – that is enough for him.

Lukas: It was an excellent suggestion by my colleague to expand the range of Mr K's nightly memories in a positive way, but compulsive thoughts cannot be overcome by gentle means. The "dreamland" associated with inner peace and relaxation as a spiritual refuge works best with "ordinary" sleep disturbances, which are caused by stressful reminiscences of the day's events. However, confronting compulsive patterns requires active defiance in the form of overt ridicule. Just as solid cliffs cannot be broken up with hammer and chisel, but only with dynamite, so the power of compulsive thoughts can only be broken with the help of paradoxical intention.

People who do not suffer from these disorders have no idea how powerful the mental forces at work actually are. They can't imagine that people under the control of their own compulsive impulses would make their own lives into a living hell. Nor can they understand that these compulsive impulses sweep like a hurricane over even intelligent people and practically paralyse their rational minds. It is incomprehensible to them that people would surrender their wills to imaginary fears. If, on the other hand, one listens to the sufferers' accounts, the full destructiveness of the compulsion can be recognised. They insist that they *must, and must continue*. On Sundays they must add up all their shopping receipts meticulously. They must change their underwear every two hours in case they are infected with bacteria. They must open just-sealed packages to check the carefully packed contents for any broken glass. They must not step on dark stones on the sidewalk because they are harbingers of misfortune. They must wrap the corners of tables and chairs in cloth in case they bite into them in a flight of delusion... I have heard this and much more in my own practice.

After at most a quarter of an hour of conversation, I no longer tolerated the word "must". Patients had to change their choice of vocabulary in homage to the truth. They had to admit: "*I wrongly believe... that I must add up my receipts, repack my packages...*" This does not (yet) heal them, but because speaking is an expression of thought, correcting the way one speaks has an effect on the way one thinks. It also increases patients' motivation to distance themselves from what they *incorrectly believe*. Who wants to be cheated? The "impostor" who had initiated them into the dark belief could then be identified with ease – however "Mr Compulsion" was metaphorically personified and parodied in the ensuing intervention.

When Marus Aurelius wrote 1900 years ago that "the happiness of your life depends on the quality of your thoughts"[8], he was probably not thinking of obsessive-compulsive disorders, but if he *had* been, he would have hit the nail on the head.

Schönfeld: After six months, Mr K asks for another appointment. Because it is the only day I can offer at short notice, he comes on his 65th birthday – so great is his despair. For weeks he has been unsettled by a dread of going to bed. His sleeping problem has become worse. Now he "must" list all the top tennis players at night along with all of their match results. He "must" know the exact days and dates of all their tournament victories. Moreover, if he ever hears any significant numbers during the day, he "must" recite them at night. These now include the lottery numbers broadcast on television, and election results from a mayoral election in a nearby city. He has always had an excellent memory for numbers, but now when he is no longer sure about today's figures for the stock market index, he "must" get up, turn on the lights, go into the next room and look through his carefully organised newspapers until he has found them. If he cannot find them, he tosses and turns sleeplessly in bed. This is why he spends the day writing page-long lists of figures, for example about the results of the latest political polls in Great Britain, the price of oil, or the number of refugees in capsized boats, and takes these lists with him to bed. If he can't remember a number, he can find it on one of his scribbled lists. Sometimes he can then fall asleep peacefully, but his relief is short, because he will soon be plagued by another question. What were the results in the Grand Slam when A and B played together? His torment has no end. "This is no kind of life," he complains. "I can't take it anymore!"

---

[8] From the 2016 quotation calendar published by the health resort of Bad Vöslau in Lower Austria.

It is time to speak plainly to him. I inform my patient about the danger and the growth of compulsive thoughts and the fact that they can be eliminated by welcoming them with humour. But the most important lesson is this: he *is* not his compulsive thoughts, he only *has* them! He is a healthy spiritual person (!), and now we should personify the pathological tendency that he *has*, so that he – like a tennis professional – can bravely face his (inner) opponent. Who is this annoying opponent, this "Mr Compulsion"? Well, as Mr K describes him, he is a rotten blackmailer who walks around holding a

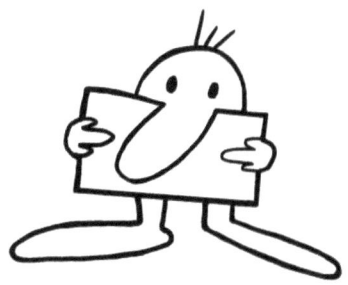 bright red placard that says: "if you can't recite the lottery numbers, you can't sleep!" He is a shabby little gnome who tries to get attention by means of threats. Intimidation is his method, and he has already won many a match with Mr K using this trick. But he can turn the tables. It is up to Mr K alone how he reacts to this insidious little dwarf and his ridiculous placard. He can put down his racquet and answer: "Of course, my dear Mr Compulsion, I am always at your service. I will immediately go and find all the numbers you ask me for!" However, he can also hit the ball back by replying: "If you're stupid enough not to know the numbers, that's *your* bad luck. I won't tell you!"

We talk more about the crucial fact that Mr K has *a choice*. Mr K can do nothing about the fact that he has this horrible opponent living in his soul. Unfortunately, this is the result of his innate predispositions. But whether or not he will allow himself to do the things that have occurred to him is *his* decision. He does not have to capitualate, he does not have to allow himself to be blackmailed – he can demonstrate with a mocking smile who is in charge. Blackmailers can only be disempowered if you don't give them what they want – *and bravely stand up to their threats*. So what does Mr Compulsion threaten him with? A wakeful night? OK. Now he can deftly parry the threat:

"You know what, I'll have plenty of time to sleep when I'm dead. Until then, I will enjoy the cuddly warmth of my duvet, stretch myself out comfortably and dream away, undisturbed by worries. I would only miss out if I slept..."

We practice "defensive strokes" to counter the insistent pressure of the blackmailer and his garish placard, which has been so effective thus far. In the future, this placard will be transformed into a humorous exchange with its bearer: "You stupid little gnome, you simply can't remember numbers, but you don't have to come begging to me about it; I'll throw all the numbers in the bin. If you want to go get them, feel free. But take care that the lid doesn't shut on you, otherwise you'll have to sit inside with all the smelly rubbish!" These little jokes amuse Mr K and he becomes increasingly bold in harassing his opponent: "If you want to visit my apartment again, you'll have to fill out ten blue application forms to apply for permission... and before you talk to me, you'll have to brush your teeth properly." At last, Mr K gave a carefree laugh. A big step towards a successful therapeutic outcome.

We agree that from now on he will never again allow himself to be sent off to his newspaper rack by the puny gnome. He will destroy all the numbers he has floating around in his apartment. For years, he has allowed himself to be meaninglessly tormented; at the age of 65 a new "compulsion-free" era will begin. *This* wil be his best birthday present: he will never again make himself ridiculous in front of Mr Compulsion, but rather, *he will make Mr Compulsion ridiculous*.

Lukas: It is a well-established rule to meet patients where they are or have their emotional roots. Mr K has a deeply-rooted enthusiasm for tennis, so it was a wise move to explain the dialectic of fate and freedom to him using the metaphor of a tennis match. His opponent's shots are "fate", and he can't control how the ball arrives. In this, we are just as powerless as the sufferer who is on the receiving end of his fears or compulsive thoughts. *Why* one's opponent plays a certain shot is just as secondary in a tennis match. The important thing is how you react as the ball heads towards you. Our freedom is in the moves we carry out *ourselves*. It is in our awareness and understanding, in the graceful movements of our arms and hands, in our commitment to fair play, in our joy in the game. A veteran like Mr K could easily be initiated into this secret. He understood: taking compulsive thoughts seriously is like standing still. Giving in to compulsive thoughts is the same as resigning the match. It means perpetual defeat. At 65 years of age, he was tired of this.

If a specialist compares my colleague's two case studies, something will immediately stand out. Mr Ks compulsive thoughts are atypical in one way. Most sufferers of obsessive-compulsive illnesses are mainly afraid of personal failure in the form of possible *guilt*. With Ms J, this fear was apparent. However, the fear can be hidden, for example, compulsive washing may be the result of a morbid fear of bacteria. This fear is often exacerbated by the horrible idea of possibly infecting other people. Or a compulsion to add up shopping receipts may be motivated by a fear of having cheated someone out of their money. A great fear for one's own self and its well-being – as with Mr K, who is worried about his sleep – is more common in cases of anxiety disorder than in cases of obsessive-compulsive disorder.

Perhaps, however, this patient also had latent feelings of guilt, namely about whether he was really the right person to train a youth team. The youths are very impressionable: they look for role models, imitating their idols and the behaviour of their leaders. This is a great responsibility, which requires sufficient mental stability to endure. We would like to trust that Mr K has striven to achieve this stability *not least* because of his influence on his team.

The doctor and philosopher Frankl described fear and compulsion as the two most fundamental clinical phenomena because they correspond to the two basic human possibilities of freedom and responsibility.

"Only a free being can be afraid... [Publisher's note: Frankl is referring not to physiological fear, but to a fear of bad decisions] and only a responsible being can be guilty. From this, it follows that a being who is granted freedom and responsibility is condemned to the possibility of fear and guilt."[9]

Schönfeld: When Mr K comes back a week later, he has sensational news. After his last session, he destroyed all the sheets of numbers, he did not get up at night all week to look up any numbers he had forgotten, and the great surprise was that he fell asleep without difficulty every night! I am very happy for him, and I ask what has helped him so greatly. Indeed, what is it? The method of paradoxical intention. Mr K has personified his number obsession as a weak, old wrinkled Mr Gnome, and now always responds to him cheekily. When Mr Gnome asked him about the tennis results in the club, he was answered: "Why don't you go down to the club yourself and ask!" In response to another urgent request from the Mr Gnome, Mr K replied that the lottery numbers had already been buried in the landfill. His witty and lighthearted responses saved him. His compulsive thoughts were immediately gone.

Sometimes a few numbers slip through his mind at night, but that is allowed. What is forbidden is only to dwell on them, because this means that Mr Gnome is unwellcomely butting in again. And that is strictly forbidden. Where are his ten completed application forms? No permission will be granted without them!

We breeze through the therapy session, and there is no further trace of Mr K's irrational fears. Of course, I prepare him for the fact that Mr Gnome is not yet dead, despite his decrepitude, and could reappear quite unexpectedly. Mr K promises to be vigilant. Besides, he says, he could use something to laugh about every so often...

---

[9] Viktor E. Frankl, Theorie und Therapie der Neurosen, UTB Ernst Reinhardt, Munich, 2007, p. 150.

He is right: laughter is healthy and lifts you up! However, you do not have to experience psychic problems to have a good laugh sometimes!

Dealing with Feelings of Guilt

Lukas: No one likes to deal with the topic of guilt, because no one likes to own up to mistakes and omissions. When people deal with this topic in their daily lives, it usually involves assigning blame to *other people*. It is quite common to ask who is to blame for any problems or misfortunes, and to complain about the allegedly guilty parties. The question, on the other hand, of what *I myself* could have done better and could still do better, is rarely asked.

Nevertheless, people are aware that they have personal shortcomings, and from time to time many brave people make an attempt to address their weaknesses. The successes achieved are not spectacular, but they do exist. With considerable effort, it is possible to rid oneself of bad habits, to learn from mistakes and to raise one's own ethical standards slightly. Looking at the present course of human history, one could find reasons to doubt this. But it must be remembered that in cosmic terms, our species has just emerged from its cradle and is still stuttering along the path of Cain and Abel. Decisive collective change will probably take longer than we can imagine.

But let us stick to the individual. As long as people are conscious, and have reached a certain stage of maturity, they possess a freedom of choice that we should not underestimate. We should certainly not try to explain it away with pseudo-scientific arguments. It is dangerous to create a concept of the human being as an automaton fed with selective information and reacting accordingly. In the 20th century, psychoanalysis made human behaviour seem "automatic". In the psychoanalytic view, negative childhood experiences mixed with strong repressed drives would lead inexorably to negative behaviour. The blame for this was removed from the shoulders of the "guilty" and attributed to their circumstances of life. In the 21st century, medical discussions allude to genetic programming and physiological brain processes. It is quite simple: if there is no freedom of will, there is no guilt. Then all people, perpetrators and victims alike, without exception – are victims.

It is obvious that this conclusion does not serve us well. That is why we will work with the logotherapeutic concept of the human being, according to which a human being always possesses freedom and responsibility, although of course not to an unlimited extent. Nor does it deny that there are restrictions to freedom and responsibility associated with illness or age. Nevertheless, in accordance with the common sense of justice shared by practically all peoples on earth, logotherapy affirms the existence of free will. This individual freedom to make decisions, and the responsibility for the decisions made, then imply that such decisions can also be wrong, unjust, cruel, or may produce suffering. The individual may realize these consequences in advance, but it is often only in retrospect that they become clear.

This brings us to an important distinction. It makes a big difference whether someone grasps the dubious nature of a decision in *advance* or in *retrospect*. The penalty in law for an illegal act also depends on this. If an individual knows in advance that the decision he or she is about to make will have negative consequences, then these consequences are accepted as part of the decision. In contrast, if one acts in good faith in an attempt to do the right thing, and negative consequences follow, then they cannot be said to have been intended.

Because logotherapy is a meaning-centred form of psychotherapy that places the question of meaning at the centre of its theory and practice, it holds that *genuine (existential) guilt requires both free-*

dom of choice and awareness of meaning. Freedom of choice, because one cannot be guilty if one had no choice. For example, a driver who loses consciousness while driving, causing an accident, cannot be blamed for the accident. This behaviour was not chosen and could not be controlled, so the accident could not have been avoided, however unfortunate its consequences were. Something similar applies to awareness of meaning. If it is not present, there can be no offence against meaning. For then there is no awareness of a meaningful alternative. A demolition expert, for example, who does not know that a hiking group has strayed into the blasting area despite clear warning signs, cannot be blamed if the hikers are injured when a blast is triggered. There was no meaningful reason to delay the blast. Accordingly, the logotherapeutic definition of guilt may be formulated as follows: *(genuine) guilt is a (free) choice against (recognised) meaning.*.

Why does logotherapy talk of "genuine" or "existential" guilt? This needs to be explained in more detail. People also suffer from unnecessary guilt, or more precisely, from something that is not guilt at all, at least not *their* guilt, but rather an unfortunate circumstance. They suffer from an unfortunate circumstance, in which either freedom of choice or awareness of meaning or both have been lacking. If, for example, the accident caused by the unconscious driver or the blast initiated by the demolition expert resulted in loss of human life, these "guiltless originators" may well reproach themselves, and these *unjustified reproaches* may hang like a cloud over the rest of their lives. There is nothing wrong with mourning the dead; every human is worthy to be mourned. But inappropriate feelings of guilt should not be allowed to prevail in these cases.

To repeat: the feelings of guilt that plague a person can be justified or unjustified, rational or irrational. They can come from an awareness of responsibility that suggests a wrong decision has been made. But they can also be the erroneous product of an oversensitive psyche that is not commensurate with its – possibly only supposed –

inadequacy. As any psychiatrist who has worked with clinically depressed or obsessive-compulsive people knows very well, feelings of guilt can even be symptoms of a mental health disorder. In such cases, feelings of guilt often testify to nothing but a disturbed mind, or at any rate, they may not indicate that the person affected is at fault, as they imagine in their delusional fantasies.

To further complicate this situation, there exist mixed forms of guilt. Freedom of choice and awareness of meaning can be partially absent, but not enough to absolve one of all guilt. Perhaps the driver who collapsed in the car could have noticed his unsatisfactory state of health in the days before the accident. Perhaps an immediate visit to the doctor would have helped. Or perhaps the doctor would have forbidden him to drive. Sufficient reflection may reveal a grey area in which there was an unused *space of freedom*. In other situations, information might have been available that would have increased the *awareness of meaning*. Perhaps the demolition expert could have checked with local hiking groups to see if any hikes had been planned in the area. Perhaps a siren or a small test firing would have driven any wanderers out of the danger zone. Many unfortunate circumstances invite questions like this in retrospect. But human freedom is not omnipotence, and human knowledge is not omniscience, so we must humbly acknowledge that in every moment of our existence we can only act in accordance with our "best knowledge and conscience", which does not guarantee that good outcomes will always result from our good intentions. "The intention is ours, the effect is God's," was Frankl's wise comment. Unfortunately, tragic effects cannot always be prevented, even with the best intentions.

Let us turn now to the practice of a psychotherapist, particularly a logotherapist. Patients and clients describe the torment caused by their feelings of guilt. Are they confused? Or is the remorse that gnaws at them genuine? How can we relieve their suffering? Below, my colleague reports on an intervention from her own practice.

Schönfeld: "I may be to blame for the death of a child," says my new patient right at the beginning of our session. Mrs L is 43 years old, a petite woman, and tells me with a gentle voice about the hideous thoughts that are oppressing her. She is a care worker and discovered her love for severely disabled children early in life. She quickly found a job in a home for disabled children. In the home, the most severely disabled children are organised into groups of ten; they all require constant care. Mrs L loves her job and enjoys being with the disabled children who mean so much to her.

Our conversation is about little Eva. She was five years old, blind, confined to a wheelchair, and could only utter low sounds. In recent months, the girl had repeatedly suffered from a high fever. On one occasion, the fever had been the result of a cold, but not the other times. Severely disabled children sometimes have a high fever that doctors cannot explain. Through these difficult months, Eva had sometimes almost died. By the summer, however, it finally looked as if she was on a path to recovery. There was no more fever.

Because it was going to be a hot August day, they had decided to go out to enjoy the cool morning air with some of the children. Mrs L pushed Eva's wheelchair through the small green park around the children's home. Other carers were with her, joking with the children – when suddenly Eva's wheelchair fell over. In the previous weeks heavy rain had washed out some of the paths and left little trenches. Mrs L, chatting happily with the others, had overlooked one of these ruts, and one of the wheels had fallen into it. The wheelchair had fallen over, and Eva had fallen to the ground, screaming in horror. Mrs L immediately picked up the little girl, pressed her to her chest, ran back into the house and hurried to the doctor's room. Eva was crying, but she only had a few little scratches on her arm, which were quickly treated with a plaster. However, the shock of the sudden fall may have been greater than the actual injuries. Eva was professionally looked after and settled with soothing words, she relaxed and soon went to sleep in her little bed. Mrs L sat with her for a long time, the little girl was breathing calmly and regularly.

In the afternoon, the fever returned. Her parents came and stayed with her, as they did most days. Although the fever increased steadily until evening, the parents were convinced that Eva was better off in the medically well-equipped home with 24-hour care than in a clinic. They refused to allow her to be taken to a hospital. They agreed that they did not want life-extending measures should her state of health become critical.

At midnight that same day, Eva died, feverish, but calm and secure in the arms of her parents. Despite the pain of losing their beloved daughter, the parents were able to deal with Eva's death in peace. They had known for a long time that Eva did not have good prospects for survival, so they were mentally prepared for the end. This was not the case for Mrs L. Could the accident in the morning have precipitated Eva's death? Had the shock caused the return of the fever in the poor girl? If the wheelchair hadn't fallen over, would the child still be alive? No one can answer these questions. But they have been eating away at Mrs L ever since. *Is she responsible for Eva's death?*

Lukas: People have different character dispositions and develop these dispositions in different ways. Character dispositions are neutral in themselves and can be used for both positive and negative purposes. A criminal instinct, for example, can be used to pursue a criminal career, but it can be used just as well to hunt down criminals in the role of an inspector or commissioner. The same applies to an innate disposition to boldness or shyness. Boldness can lead to insensitivity and a lack of moral awareness, but it can also produce composure and resolution. Shyness can cause inhibitions and overscrupulousness, but it can also make a person careful and cautious. Ultimately, less depends on our predispositions themselves than on how we use and control them.

Patients like Mrs L undoubtedly belong to the category of people who are insecure, anxious, want to do everything right and tend to worry too much. A carer with a more robust mental constitution would probably have "signed off" Eva's death as an act of fate and turned back to the other children in the home. But that is not to say that Mrs L is completely wrong or that her response is pathological. She has a particularly sensitive conscience, which should be seen as a good thing. She has an enormous appreciation for children who are severely disabled and disadvantaged in life, and one can only marvel at this. She is a decent and kind person, who deserves respect. The only danger that she has to be careful to avoid is that she might succumb to perfectionism, or that she might recriminate herself whenever she does not succeed perfectly. An excessively loud voice of conscience (hyperacusis) is just as contrary to meaning as a muffled one. A healthy sense of responsibility lies exactly between these two extremes.

Schönfeld: We review what happened once again. No doubt the moment of the fall took its toll on Eva. But it is unlikely that the accident affected the girl so much that it was responsible for the return of her fever. However, one cannot say anything for certain in the case of severely disabled children. One thing is certain, however: after her fall, Eva was cared for and treated immediately in the optimal way. She was surrounded with affection and love, comforted and protected. Eva could not express herself in words, but the fact that she fell asleep so soon proves how quickly she became calm and relaxed again.

Mrs L tells me more about Eva. Two years ago, she had come into the home as a screaming and writhing bundle. In the home, with the help of medically professional, self-sacrificing care that the parents could never have provided to the same extent, she made a great deal of progress. She learned how to smile for the first time. She clearly enjoyed her life. How wonderful! "She would have loved to have lived longer," says Mrs L. "Am I to blame for her death?"

Together we consider how guilt can be assessed from a logotherapeutic perspective (which goes beyond a legal or religious context). In order to speak of guilt, two things must be present: 1. a freely willed decision, and 2. a clear awareness of meaning. Whatever one willingly and intentionally strives for, decides for, one is also responsible for. Everything good that one accomplishes, and everything bad that one brings into the world. But to be responsible, one must also know whether what one has chosen is contrary to meaning. Whether it will create suffering. Whether it will darken someone's life. Whether it will create burdens for other people. This intention is a prerequisite for genuine guilt.

Mrs L understands these criteria, and we apply them to the unfortunate event during her walk. Mrs L is very clear: she certainly never wanted the accident to happen. As she had strolled through the park, joking with the children and colleagues, she had had no idea that the ground had become so furrowed. So had she made a deliberate choice "contrary to meaning"? She admitted that she had not. We hold this point firmly in mind. It remains true, even if the child had been made more susceptible to the fever by the fall. It remains true even if, in fact, the child died sooner than would have been the case if the accident had not happened,

Lukas: Because Mrs L is not only a sensitive but also a clever woman, she understands that there is something between guilt and innocence called "negligence". As my colleague correctly argued, this has to do with *knowledge*, with an *awareness* of possibly having acted contrary to meaning. One can increase this knowledge by paying careful attention (or by actively obtaining information). For example, if Mrs L had paid more attention to the ground and less to her conversation, she might have noticed the large furrows in time. It is easy to speculate about such things in retrospect. In life, we all act a bit carelessly or negligently on countless occasions, and nothing bad happens. We may escape disaster by a thread a thousand times. But on the thousandth time, we may be unlucky.

It is therefore good to acknowledge openly that being human involves weakness and inadequacy, and that it is almost impossible to avoid all (non-intentional) mistakes and failures. We can only *try* to be mindful and accept the occasional disasters not as "personal guilt", but as "intrinsic shortcomings of the human species". There is something else we can do: nothing prevents us from taking the initiative to do good things and use our energies for the benefit of other people and the environment. Logotherapy offers the excellent suggestion of counterbalancing guilt and negligence with positive inner attitudes and deliberate good deeds. If, intentionally or unintentionally, we have caused something bad to happen, this provides us with a good reason to put something especially loving and constructive on the other side of the scale to balance the account of our lives.

Schönfeld: As is usual in logotherapy, I direct the patient's attention away from her own ego. Her significance in the story is only in fourth place. The most important people in the story are Eva and her two parents. We think about these three people. The parents knew that their child would not live long. The doctor had explained to them that the fever attacks would gradually get worse and Eva's chances of survival would continuously decrease. Her father and mother had come to terms with this, and they were grateful that the home enabled Eva to enjoy the time remaining to her. They were able to accept the death of their daughter, with great sadness, but without strife or despair. Und Eva? Until her death, she was enveloped in a network of daily care, and lifted up in constant love. Unfortunately, not all of the children in our world can say that about themselves.

I ask Mrs L what Eva would say now, if she could listen to our conversation. "My life was beautiful in spite of everything," suggests

Mrs L. For the child had died content, despite severe illness and fever. So many people have to live year after year in miserable surroundings and in solitude. I ask Mrs L again: what would Eva say if she could be here with us? Mrs L says spontaneously, "She would spread her arms wide and turn her big blind eyes towards us. She always did that when she knew that someone was there". And what would Mrs L do? She would ask for forgiveness. Then what would Eva do next?

Mrs L shakes her head, perplexed. I make a suggestion. Perhaps Eva would think: Everyone should rue their actions! I am dead; now let others suffer! Mrs L rejects this idea firmly. Eva would never say anything like that, that is not like her at all. I suggest instead that Eva might think: "At least Mrs L should suffer immense feelings of guilt, that would make me happy!" "No, no!" Mrs L interrupts me, "Never! Eva would never think that!" I try something else. Perhaps Eva would think: "I do not want my death to cause great unhappiness in the life of Mrs L!"

We consider this possibility for a long time. Mrs L is certain that it is not compatible with the sweet nature of this child to be the cause of terrible sorrow. It is not acceptable to make her the cause of human misfortune. No, the girl should not be burdened with the charge of having upset Mrs L's mental balance with her death. What traces of Eva, what memories of her should be allowed to endure? A gnawing, irrational sense of guilt? Or rather, her outstretched arms and her smile? Is it possible to honour the memory of Eva by burdening it with endless self-reproach?

Mrs L is silent for a while, then takes a deep breath and asks: "But does this not let me off too easily?"

Lukas: At this point, let us interject an observation that is well confirmed by experience. Of course, people can speak to a dead person. In doing so, they do not speak to the corpse in the coffin, but to the *person* they knew. "Where" this person is now is beyond our comprehension, because space and time are annihilated by death, but as living beings we cannot think outside space and time. Nevertheless, one can imagine an inner dialogue with a dead person, and at moments of special spiritual closeness to the person, one can even imagine answers that are felt as intensely as if one had received them "from the void". The interesting thing is that in all reports of such "imaginary dialogues" (Fabry) the answers received are merciful, understanding, and mild, as if in death only what is good counts. It is too glib to interpret this phenomenon as mere wishful thinking. Even in the case of "imaginary dialogues" with former enemies and aggressors, listeners report only benevolent responses. It is therefore not surprising that Mrs L, despite her self-critical nature, affirms without hesitation that Eva wishes her only the best and does not want her to torment herself with feelings of guilt.

This is how we can answer the question of whether Mrs L is "let off too easily" by the comforting logotherapeutic arguments of my colleague. There is only *one* person who can absolve her from all of her (imagined?) guilt, Eva herself. If Mrs L is convinced that Eva would not wish her any unhappiness, then *the authority on the matter has spoken.*

Schönfeld: In our next session, we continue our philosophical debate. Errors made, mistakes committed, lapses of attention may also have positive consequences. One should pay attention to this as well. For example, Mrs L's deep remorse has made her into a new person. Her unending regret that she overturned the child's wheelchair in a rut is a guarantee that she will never make the same mistake again. Other disabled children will benefit from this. Once again, Mrs L's attention is directed away from herself. What about the other children she cares for? Can she really care for them properly if part of her is constantly preoccupied with self-accusations about Eva? Brooding over Eva's death diverts her attention from her current care duties. Would the other children in the home not benefit if Mrs L converted her repentance and self-reproach into a determination to take particularly good care of those who depend on her?

Mrs L still sometimes finds it difficult to forgive herself. Eva's parents do not blame her, Eva does not blame her, she is the only one who accuses herself so harshly. I tell her about Viktor Frankl, who asserted that it is not for us to set conditions and ask questions of life, but it is life that sets us conditions and asks us questions. Mrs L wanted to demand from life that she could live out her days without ever making a serious mistake; she wanted to allow herself only small errors. Now, however, what life is asking her is this: "In an unfortunate moment, you had an unintentional lapse, which may or may not have done harm – how will you deal with it?" Yes, how? Meaningfully? Or not meaningfully?

I play out possibilities with her. One possible answer she could give to life is: "I will never be happy again." This answer is possible, but is it meaningful? It is not, because this answer increases the suffering in the world. What is a possible answer that does not increase suffering? Perhaps an answer that even reduces suffering. We collect together possible answers. Mrs L comes back to the other children in the home. She must not pay any less attention to them. She examines her heart: her feelings for these children have not changed. She still takes care of them lovingly. Is this perhaps already an optimal answer to the question life is asking her? What if she could say to herself: "I've been a bit careless – it's time to add something good and useful to the wheelchair accident... something I *wouldn't have automatically done anyway*."

This idea fascinates her. She thinks for a while, then she has an idea. In addition to care duties, there are more and more technical medical tasks that need to be done in the home. Most of the time these tasks make her feel flustered and insecure, so she avoids them as much as possible. But that's not good, she admits. This would be an area of her work in which she could improve her skills and lessen the workload of her colleagues. It would also be a very good opportunity for "reparation": in the past she was "not completely competent" – in the future she could be "a bit more competent". These technical medical tasks are also important for the children in the home, so why not extend her service of love in this way? Mrs L decides to summon up all her courage and says: "I'll do it – I'll perfect my skills so that I can perform the technical tasks that I've been avoiding so far!"

Lukas: The approach of logotherapy is not to minimise genuine guilt with psychological "excuses" (as is often done in counselling), but to offer conscious reparation. Human conscience is a sensitive instrument that is difficult to deceive. However, it can be appeased by means of reparations offered with clear intention and honest effort. Surprisingly, reparations do not have to benefit the injured parties or things. Of course, if the damage can still be repaired, this has priority over all other actions. But unfortunately this is not always the case, as in Eva's story. The voice of conscience calls us not to give up in this case, but to "make amends" in some other area of the world. There always exist dark corners of the world in need of a shining light, should we need to turn to them. There is no more beautiful and noble response to guilt than to use it to motivate new acts of human kindness. If this is combined with a lasting purification and transformation of the self, this is undoubtedly *superior*.

One of my former patients once ended a tragic account of her life with the words: "Everything that has become of me is all because I brought guilt upon myself as a young woman. The knowledge of this guilt changed me for the better. I couldn't make up for what I did, but all the good I did later, was only the result of this knowledge."[10] Isn't this an exemplary answer to the question life had asked her: "You made a mistake...what now?"

---

[10] Elisabeth Lukas, *Auch dein Leiden hat Sinn, Logotherapeutischer Trost in der Krise*, Herder, Freiburg/Br., 1994, p. 140.

There is a big difference, however, between my former patient (who was guilty of a crime of passion) and my colleague's patient. On the basis of this report, I personally do not believe that Mrs L. is guilty of anything at all. On the contrary, she is far more committed to the severely disabled children than her job would require. Nor is she a careless woman – her tendency is to be overcareful. Unfortunately, however, she is being controlled by a primal fear, and it will be a while before she will be able to regain her basic trust. This primal fear is constantly whispering in her ear: "Perhaps you are still guilty." This is why my colleague correctly brought the therapeutic concept of reparation into play, despite the fact that the guilt was merely imagined and probably non-existent. This achieved two things: 1. some resistance is offered to the primal fear, and 2. the primal fear reveals itself clearly at last.

Primal fear wears many veils: fear of this and fear of that. You could make a mistake, you could embarrass yourself, you could be criticised, accused, laughed at, you could lose your status, your reputation, your health, your job...so it goes on and on. Primal fear always thinks of something. It is never short of threatening visions. Thus it immediately attacks Mrs L's bold plans in order to spoil them for her. Bold plans are a dangerous thing for fears.

Schönfeld: Mrs L soon loses heart again. She would like to learn how to perform the technical medical tasks in the home, but how can she overcome the nervousness and panic attacks that usually afflict her when she tries to do so?

I can help her with this. For early humans, fear was an important protective factor. When danger was present, it increased pulse rate and muscle tension, pumped adrenaline into the blood and produced greater alertness. This allowed early humans to fight against wild animals or flee from them, or to climb up trees. Similar psychophysical reactions take place in us when we are exposed to danger. This even occurs if the danger exists only in our minds. For example,

118

because Mrs L associates the difficult technical medical tasks with a danger of failure, attempting them causes an adrenaline rush, and her muscles begin to shake. She has to choose between fight or flight. Flight means running away and fighting back by refusing to perform the task. This has been her strategy so far. But she could also fight. But how do you fight an exaggerated fear? I reveal a megaweapon: *humour*. It is even worse for fear than courage, because it annihilates fear completely.

My suggestion is to smile and mock the fear by saying, "What a welcome burst of energy! I can put you to work making sure that I can concentrate well on my new task! I want to start right away and solve this problem optimally – and you will help me!" Mrs L warms to this approach right away. She wants to try it. "If it gives me an energy boost, then bring on the anxiety!" I am pleased that Mrs L accepts my suggestion. It would be wonderful if something good would come out of the wheelchair accident, in that Mrs L would be braver in overcoming her difficulties with the dreaded technical tasks. Eva would be proud to have been the cause of this development.

A month later, Mrs L has a relapse. The thought that she might have precipitated Eva's death has taken hold of her again. We discuss the wheelchair accident again point by point. It is still the case that the doctor can not say anything with certainty. The only thing that is absolutely certain is that the girl died peacefully, cocooned in love and security.

Lukas: Empathy is truly a divine gift. People who can empathise with others and perceive their state of mind are always very socially minded, and unlikely to behave like a bull in a china shop. They are considerate and tolerant of their fellow human beings, and do not judge them for their failures. While it is not true that "to understand all is to forgive all", as some over-optimistically assert, empathy makes it possible to smooth over many misunderstandings before they develop into full-blown conflicts.

Empathy is a special ability to mirror another person's feelings. This makes it possible to discern what another person is feeling, and to conclude what is going on in them on the basis of one's own feelings. Empathetic people are instinctively aware, for example, that insults are hurtful – for themselves and thus for the people they interact with. The parallels they are able to draw between themselves and others immediately causes them to put the brakes on any hurtful behaviour. However, as in all things, there is another side to the coin. Making conclusions about other people based on one's own feelings can lead to interpretations that miss the mark, in spite of empathetic skills. Psychoanalysis refers to these misinterpretations as "projections". It may be that one projects one's own feelings onto someone else in a similar situation, but they experience it differently. Projection is often done unconsciously.

The persistence with which Mrs L's experience with Eva in the park is mentally associated with the outbreak of fever later in the afternoon suggests to an expert that projection is taking place. We have discovered that Mrs L is prone to anxiety. If she had fallen out of a moving vehicle herself, she would have been extremely startled. She knows herself well enough to suspect that it would have taken a while to recover from such a trauma. Even if her injuries had been minimal, it would have had a significant effect on her for days, or even weeks. In any case, certainly for the next few hours. Mrs L therefore concludes that it must have been this way for Eva as well.

This conclusion is not justified. Disabled children do not simulate recovery. When Eva stopped crying, calmed down and fell asleep easily, we can only assume that, for her, everything was right with the world again. We can also assume that, as a result of her blindness, the girl was used to sudden, unexpected contact – not harsh shocks like falling to the ground, but at least bumping into the corners and edges of unseen objects. There is nothing in Mrs L's account to suggest that Eva would have been seriously distressed by the last afternoon of her life. *The Person who was really distressed was not Eva, but Mrs L.* Nor is there any evidence to suggest that Eva's final attack of fever was different from the previous attacks, which, according to Mrs L herself, and in the opinion of the doctor, all occurred without any external trigger, except in one case of a cold (and this was *not a psychological trigger*).

Mrs L will eventually have to realise that her own distress about Eva's death has taken her so much by surprise that she has succumbed to panic and invented a baseless theory of guilt. However, I would like to stress that she should dial back the agitation and anxiety very carefully, so that she can remain the lovable, empathetic woman she is, who has a job for which she is extremely well-suited and which she performs admirably.

Schönfeld: Mrs L is at a crossroads. She cannot avoid having the thought of possibly being responsible for Eva's death. But she can choose how to respond to it. She can give into it and enter voluntarily into a permanent state of agony and regret. This will rob her of the strength she needs for her work. In the long run, the children in the home will perceive her distress, for, like all children, they are finely attuned to moods. This would place Eva's memory in a permanent shadow. There is, however, an alternative path open to Mrs L – she can refuse to play along with the thought. She can stubbornly and consistently refuse to give space to the thought of her possible guilt. She can declare an end to brooding and increasing suffering in the world. It will be a difficult path – there is not much pleasure in this kind of resistance. But it will work if she knows what she is doing it for: putting a stop to the brooding would be a fitting tribute to Eva's memory. Only by putting an end to these thoughts will she be able to devote her efforts to the other children in the home, who need her undivided attention.

Mrs L has to decide between these two paths. She alone can determine which of them she will take.

Weeks later, we say goodbye. Mrs L says that she has been working on the "technical medical stuff" in the past weeks. She checks the machines and looks after the equipment, and her colleagues are grateful. Excellent! This is part of the good legacy that is growing up around the memory of Eva. The home has acquired a caregiver who is skilled in the use of technical medical equipment.

Mrs L also tells me that a new child called Stefan has arrived at the home. He is nine months old, but he looks like a newborn. The boy was born lifeless. He was resuscitated after ten minutes, but he has never been able to breathe on his own. With heavy hearts the parents had decided to send their little Stefan to the home to receive palliative care. His mother sits at his bedside every day.

Mrs L has made a clear decision about her path. She knows that for the sake of this child alone, she needs to get rid of her remaining unjustified feelings of guilt. She now needs all her strength and presence of mind for Stefan! For him, and for all the other children. These severely disabled children all have serious health problems – and yet they are more protected than most children on Earth. I say to Mrs L: "There seems to me that there is more love in your care home than anywhere else." I am thinking of the love with which she cares for the children. She nods, but then I get a completely unexpected response. "Yes, we get so much back from these children! It is such a special place!" She is happy to work there.

I have the greatest respect for all caregivers, and especially for Mrs L. I learned a lot from her.

Dealing with Trauma

Lukas: Global trends suggest that in the future we can expect not only more heatwaves and droughts, but also more and more migrations and refugee routes. This is the logical consequence of population increase coupled with a decrease of habitable space. Just as affordable housing is increasingly difficult to find in industrial cities, it will also become increasingly difficult to find pleasant areas to live in. Millions of people will migrate from country to country in a desperate effort to escape disastrous political, climatic, and economic conditions.

Logically, an inevitable consequence is that these millions of people will be *traumatised*. People who flee from disastrous circumstances will have experienced disastrous circumstances, and undoubtedly for a long time. Circumstances must be terrifying to induce people to leave their home, their accustomed culture and their social network and venture into the unknown. For many of them, what awaits them will also be terrifying. They will be rejected and resented, and even if they are lucky enough to be taken in by another country, they will certainly *not* be offered therapy to help them deal with their trauma. They will be lucky if fortune allots them some food, blankets, tents and even a few medical supplies. The big winners in the lottery of fate might receive training or offers of work.

I mention this, because it should be clear to all of us that in the future we will have to deal with large numbers of traumatised people who will have to rebuild themselves through their own efforts or degenerate into mental wrecks. As a psychotherapist, I know what that means. But as a child of the wartime generation, I also know that people of this generation in Europe, who were burdened with similarly traumatic experiences (and also lacked therapeutic help), were able to realise their dreams in an astonishingly successful way. This should give us confidence in the veracity of Frankl's "tragic optimism", which involved the conviction that human beings are at the mercy of their physical and psychic circumstances, but *not in their spiritual capacities*. Human beings possess a power of defiance that can renew everything and enable them to rise from the ashes like a phoenix, if necessary.

The problem is that these days many people are unaware of this fact.

Schönfeld: 36 year old Mrs M comes to me because she can't sleep well and often wakes up at night. As she also sometimes has to get up at night because of her three small children, her sleep is considerably disturbed. This, however, is only the first thing she says when she explains why she has come to me. Immediately afterwards, she adds that her sleeping disorder is no surprise, because she had a terrible childhood.

While I am still considering whether I should enquire about her childhood in more detail, she is already in full flow. Her mother died shortly after her birth. Her father remarried a year later. She believes that this was mostly to provide a mother for his three young children. This however, was not successful, because her stepmother cared less for the children than for pretty clothes and luxurious living. Mrs M was also sexually abused by her uncle. A few years ago, she had a stroke. This was completely unexpected, and she nearly died. There have been a number of strokes in her maternal family, so she probably has a genetic predisposition to them. For several months, she suffered from paralysis in parts of her body, which was only over-come with physiotherapy and a lot of exercise. She now has to take strict care of her lifestyle, eat healthily and exercise regularly to minimise the chance of another stroke.

"Everything went wrong in my life – I have had so much misfortune," she laments repeatedly. She envies children who have a protected childhood – she experienced no protection. As a girl, she knew exactly what she wanted to do for a career: she wanted to run a stable. She had a deep love for horses from an early age. Her stepmother, however, ignored this wish and forced her to take a job as a supermarket apprentice. At first, she did not like the retail industry. Later she found a job in a pharmacy, which was better. She still works there, reasonably happily, though because of her children she only works three half days a week. "Everything went wrong in my life..." is her complaint.

Lukas: The theory of relativity does not just apply to physics. The evaluation of facts is also *relative* in psychology, and this evaluation is highly *subjective.*

This is why we should not try to compare two different situations of suffering. From the perspective of an African refugee who is pulled half-drowned out of the Mediterranean, Mrs M lives in a safe country, together with her husband and children, has a well-furnished apartment, a job with a good salary, healthcare and a pension, sleeps in a soft bed and does not have to worry about losing all of these comforts. The refugee might forget that the evaluation of this situation is *relative.* We must not forget this in psychotherapeutic practice. Nevertheless, we often have to correct patients' perspectives, because they are too close to misjudgments, and pave the way for mental derailments.

Thus, we must protest against Mrs M's evaluation that "everything" in her life so far has gone wrong. For example, her recovery from her stroke calls for joy and gratitude. Her three lively, healthy children are also a great gift. People who do not appreciate their gifts, or only recognise them after they have been lost, are not only unspeakably stupid, but deprive themselves of quality of life.

As patients who are suffering are often not receptive to the positive things in their lives, there is a useful trick to use with them. They are first shown what *they themselves* have succeeded in doing in a positive way, before being cautiously pointed to the positive aspects of their fate. Who will refuse genuine praise? People who are given praise are always more willing to praise others or other things than they would otherwise be.

Schönfeld: I can't agree with Mrs M. The woman in front of me has bravely overcome a serious illness. She could have complained continually and exasperated her whole family, but instead she confronted her fate bravely by undergoing a difficult rehabilitation. For this, she deserves respect! She has set her two sons and her daughter a commendable example. She could have allowed herself to be cared for by others, instead of reclaiming her own independent life.

Mrs M thinks about this and agrees. She deserves even more respect precisely *because* she did not have it easy as a child. In this situation, she did not withdraw from all social contact, nor did she become embittered. Instead, she has given her own children the secure environment for growth that she herself was denied. This deserves the highest recognition!

Mrs M is surprised at this perspective, but she says that it is true. She even adds that she is lucky in her husband. It is true that she has a really good marriage and wonderful children, she admits. And yet she is often sad because there has been so much hardship in her life. She lost her innocence too soon, she had to grow up before her time, she experienced hard years.

Then let's take a closer look at the hard things, as well as the good ones. Philosophically speaking, nothing is distributed fairly. It may well be that her childhood was more difficult than other people's childhoods. For a while, we reflect on the fact that, as humans, there are many things in which we have no choice. There is always something inevitable facing us that we would never have chosen. However, there is *one choice* that we are free to make, and that is the decision of where to focus our attention. For example, she can can choose to focus on the desolation of her past life. Alternatively, she can focus on more gratifying things: on her children, her happy marriage, the recovery from her stroke. This is her own decision, and it will determine whether her days are clouded over or bathed in soft light.

Whichever decision we make, and even if we turn our attention to the good things, the *suffering we have experienced remains suffering.* No one can take it away from us. The question is whether it continues to be merely detrimental to us or not. Persevering through suffering often enables us to develop a certain "competence of suffering" (Lukas). We develop skills that cannot develop in pleasant and comfortable phases of life. Mrs M immediately understands what I mean. Yes, she has learned to fight. If there is something in her family that has to be fought for, then it is always *her* who finds a way through it. But, she says, the price for this was too high.

Lukas: Scientists have performed numerous studies on victims of trauma. Let us first note the following: the people who have been studied have all *survived* their traumas. I emphasise this, because terrible events (earthquakes, active duty in war, etc.) can also end in the death of the individuals involved. Thus, people who have survived a trauma have experienced a degree of mercy in the midst of the inferno. Whether they appreciate their survival is up to them. The fact is, however, that life itself offers many possibilities for shaping life after trauma in individual ways. Whenever freedom opens up, the will gradually reawakens and urges one to creativity.

A further observation: no one is the same after trauma as in the "life before". Trauma changes people. In what way are they changed? This is where different spirits literally separate. If the will for revenge, hatred, anger, or strife dominates, there can be no life situation that is not overshadowed by the past. In all the rooms of the present, the trauma will always be lurking in ambush. If, on the other hand, the "will to meaning" (Frankl) dominates, the change in the individual will be the development of valuable new abilities. Suffering people are sensitised. They *know* what hurts and how much it hurts! And *because* they know this, they are particularly strongly committed to preventing the same pain from spreading to other people.

The technician who invented the first emergency call system on the German Autobahn had a son who had bled to death in an accident on the Autobahn because the ambulance arrived too late. A well-known Munich social education worker did much to confront family violence, for example initiating discussion groups for men who had lost control and committed violent acts. He was blind in one eye as a result of a blow from his father. Studies are full of examples of suffering people who have become a blessing to others. Mrs M is no exception. Instead of following her stepmother's example (a woman who was also responsible for three children), she provides the warm environment for her three children that she herself was denied. This proves that: 1. no one is forced to follow the models of behaviour they have experienced, and 2. a tragedy does not necessarily lead on to further tragedies. It can also be an opportunity for an inner triumph.

Unfortunately, Mrs M has not yet achieved her inner triumph. Her "will to meaning" is still mixed up with elements of anger and resentment, which harden her. Part of my colleague's therapeutic work will be to eliminate these elements.

Schönfeld: In our next meeting, Mrs M tells me about a family gathering that was overshadowed by the recent death of a family member. Since then, she has been thinking about death, which she narrowly escaped herself. We talk about what a good death might look like. Ideally, this would involve a full life followed by a peaceful departure.

She could not die in peace today, she says. There is too much anger burning in her. It would spoil her peace. I ask what keeps her anger burning.

It's my uncle, she explains. Her stepmother was self-centred and desirous of luxury. For this reason, she was extremely interested in the uncle (Mrs M's birth mother's brother) who had returned to Germany after living in America for many years. He drove a sports car, bought himself a holiday home on the North Sea and lived in great style. This fascinated Mrs M's stepmother, who often invited him to their house. But the uncle had little interest in her or his two nephews; he concentrated his attentions on Mrs M, who was 11 years old at the time. He spoiled her with small gifts, which Mrs M appreciated. She was starved for affection, which she had received from neither her stepmother nor her father, who had to work hard and wanted his rest in the evening. Her uncle, in contrast, had time for her. He took her to a horse farm nearby, and during the holidays she was allowed to go with him to the North Sea. This was very nice.

This happy period, however, only lasted for a short time. One evening during the holidays, her uncle suddenly appeared naked in the bathroom while she was taking a shower. She was shocked, avoided him and only reluctantly endured him touching her while they were in the car. Back home, she told her stepmother, who did not believe a word of her story. She could not believe that this elegant man could be capable of such misconduct. In the end, she was forced into sexual intercourse in the uncle's home. Mrs M remembers this terrible event clearly. She lay in bed as if frozen and did not dare to defend herself. The pain was immense. She hid the bloody panties from her stepmother – how could she have told her about *this*? Then she pretended to have a stomach ache and stayed in bed for two days. She was convinced that no one would believe her. However, the fact that she was "ill" seemed to have frightened her uncle, who of course knew what was going on. Perhaps he was afraid that his crime would be revealed. In any case, he came to visit much less often after that and eventually stayed away completely.

"No one would have believed me, no one was on my side! The man was never reported!" cried out my patient in tears.

I ask what happened to her after that. She moved away from home as soon as she was 18 years old. She shared a tiny apartment with a friend, and she had a wonderful time. Her cheery friend took her along whenever she went out. Soon both had found their first boyfriends. They lived in a completely carefree way. After a few pleasant years she met her current husband. It was love at first sight, and nothing has changed to this day.

I ask her about her first voluntary sexual encounters. She reported that she and the boys of her age were clumsy, as most young people probably are at first. With her husband, however, this had also led to a happy coexistence.

Lukas: Being raped was undoubtedly a traumatic event in this patient's life. The only small doubt in her story is of a different nature. This is the doubt about whether it is true that neither her stepmother nor her father, nor a teacher nor any other person close to the girl would have believed her if she had made the dreadful event known. But the girl did her best (feigning a stomach ache) to deceive her family. The poor child! She did not dare to defend herself from the rape, and she did not dare to report it. Instead, she suffered in silence.

If we look more closely at my patient's outcry: "No one was on my side! The man was never reported!" then it is impossible not to see the connection. No one was on her side, *because no one – apart from the perpetrator – knew anything about the deed*. The man was never reported *because no one was aware of his crime*. Poor woman! At that time, she could probably have been prevented the thing she grieves about to this day. Of course, she doesn't want to admit *this* to herself! Therefore she claims: "No one would have believed me!"

One must be careful with interpretations. Perhaps the incident would really have been swept under the carpet. But bloody panties are a pretty solid piece of evidence. Also, we only know about the child's tensions with the stepmother from the child's point of view. If we could hear the stepmother's point of view, we would certainly hear a very different story. It is certainly not easy to marry a widower with three children. This is especially true when the husband is exhausted by his job and provides little support in the complex task of looking after the children.

Although we must be careful with interpretations, *one* thing is indisputable: during the wonderful time that Mrs M spent with her friend after her 18th birthday, no one prevented her from reporting her uncle to the police. Perhaps the uncle would have denied everything, but the authorities would certainly have investigated the suspected crime, and this would have tarnished his reputation. That at least would provided some satisfaction for Mrs M.

It seems strange to me that in Mrs M's story, she used the "wonderful time" after her domestic trauma for nothing more than going out and getting to know young men. It would have been much more "wonderful" if, for example, she had revived the love of horses that she had felt from an early age. Why did she not pursue her desired profession as a horse keeper?

There are missed opportunities for meaning in every human life, and it is always difficult to admit them to oneself. The most frequently used tactic against such unwanted self-awareness is to point out the mistakes and omissions of other people. Even to blame those other people for one's own failures. It is not out of the question that Mrs M was employing this kind of distractive manoeuvre. In the anger that burns inside her, there could be a tiny grain of "anger at herself".

Schönfeld: Mrs M asks me as a specialist whether something of her childhood trauma has remained with her.

We divide up the different aspects of her human nature. Her uncle damaged her body and her psyche. This is a grave fact, which should not be ignored. However, as a *person* there is no scratch on her. The unmistakable essence of a person always remains healthy and the uncle could not touch it.

The injured girl's body has long since healed. Her psyche has healed as well. Mrs M has matured into a contented wife and mother.

For her, everything can be "good again". The same cannot be said for her uncle. His identity as a rapist will never change, it cannot be "made good". For his crime is stored in the record of truth, and even after his death truth will not become untruth.

Mrs M lets out a deep breath. And what about her stepmother? Yes, it is sad that she played her role so weakly. It is possible that she was overwhelmed by her many responsibilities. Perhaps she did not understand how it was possible that the rich and friendly uncle was more interested in an 11-year-old child than in her. It is also possible that she had a falsely idealised image of the uncle. Or that she placed hopes in him that he did not live up to. We know too little about these people to judge. What we do know, however, is that Mrs M has developed into a strong personality *despite* all her childhood suffering.

"Despite" – this proud word describes many episodes in her life. Mrs M smiles.

Lukas: My colleague has successfully woven two basic logo-therapeutic concepts into the therapeutic process.

1. Firstly, the *intactness of the person*. We are only vulnerable to injury in our body and psyche. Of course, this is quite enough vulnerability, and we may even be destroyed physically or psychically. Mrs M was severely wounded as a child, and her body's self-healing powers had to "work" to restore her to health, until, after some years, she was able to enter into a normal life full of cheerful activities and varied love affairs. Her self-healing powers were severely strained for a second time when a stroke threatened to paralyse her body and depress her psyche. Mrs M will also have needed her self-healing powers in the course of her three pregnancies.

However, in addition to these organic processes, every human being is a spiritual being. This spirit grants a human being freedom of will, awareness of meaning, the ability to shape itself and a glorious "defiance of the spirit" (Frankl), which, together with the body's self-healing powers, has enabled Mrs M to love her husband in spite of her childhood trauma and to be a good mother to her children. Although the human spirit can be impeded and even blocked by physical diseases and defects, it belongs itself to a dimension not subject to diseases and defects. It is like light. No light is emitted by a broken lamp. If the lamp can be repaired, it will produce light again. And no one will claim that light itself was broken – light remains light despite melted cables or broken switches. In the same way, Mrs M's spirit is untouched by all of her negative experiences.

2. Secondly, Mrs M was informed of the *unassailability of the past*. The past does not disappear, as we often mistakenly think. Rather, it continues to exist in eternal truth, and cannot be removed. Only what is possible but does not happen disappears (from the space of possibilities). What does happen, on the other hand, becomes history. In our case, it becomes *our history*.

In the case of Mrs M's uncle, there are events that would have been possible but did not happen that might have been shining highlights in his life story: creating the legacy of a child's paradise with the outings to the horse farm or to the North Sea. These possibilities, however, have disappeared. What actually happened has etched itself into his life story and driven away all its attractiveness.

There was a striking discussion of this point by victims of abuse at a logotherapy congress in Canada. They said that what they had suffered was "escapable". They still had and would always have the possibility to develop into decent, sensitive and cheerful people. Their circumstances were harder than those of other people, but their history still offered all these glorious possibilities. Their abusers, on the other hand, were abusers for all time – "inescapably". They might repent, they might change, but they could never escape from what they did. No power in the world (or beyond it) can remove anything from eternal truth.

133

It sounds strange, but from this perspective, the uncle is to be pitied. *He* lost his innocence, not the girl. He damaged himself and his life more than he damaged the girl. He will be "punished" infinitely longer than any earthly judgment could have punished him.

Schönfeld: All these reflections are balm to the soul of Mrs M. She admits that her constant indignation about her uncle does her no good. Unfortunately, she can no longer hold him to account, because he has since died. He lives on only as a barb in her thoughts, and these weigh on her almost every day. She knows perfectly well that she should forgive him, but she is unable to do so.

I tell her that forgiveness is a big word. It refers to a magnanimous inner attitude that one can ask for but never force. It is a miracle cure for traumatic injuries, a balm that heals jagged wounds, and an opportunity for offenders to reform themselves.

But how about starting with something smaller? How about letting go of resentment? For it should be clear on whose shoulders the burden of resentment lies: on the shoulders of the one who carries it. Mrs M understands this right away. Her resentment weighs heavily on her, as does the barb in her thoughts and the festering wounds it inflicts. Her uncle feels nothing of this! This is crazy! It is time to put an end to this farce. *But how?*

I ask her if she knows where her uncle is buried. She says she does, though she has never been to his grave. In that case, I recommend that if she is brave enough and has the time, she should go to the cemetery and visit his grave. When she is standing in front of his grave, she should recall her memories of her uncle. She should do this carefully, in case resentment overtakes her again. But she should concentrate hard, and begin by remembering everything about him that was good and kind. How he took care of her as a girl, his funny conversations, his gifts. Mrs M protests. "What? Remember the good side of this monster?" Yes, otherwise it will not work. You can't talk to a monster, but that's exactly what she needs to do. And there were some good times, pleasant hours in which he interacted with her playfully and without ulterior motives. This too belongs to the truth and must not be concealed. Even if there was only the tiniest grain of good in him, that is precisely what she needs to dig out of her memory.

She needs to stand at his grave, imagine the good interactions with him, and let an image of him arise before her. She should wait until the waves of emotion in her chest have subsided. When he is standing in front of her inner eye, she can tell him about everything: her horror as a child, her razor-sharp pain, all the resentment and anger she has carried since then. All the burdens she carries to this day should be laid out in front of him. She can even say that it would have been great to have a real friendship with him, especially since there were such promising moments between them at the beginning. And she can ask him why this friendship had to be destroyed so quickly.

He should be forced to listen to all of this. When she is finished, she might get an answer from him. For, after all, he is still "alive" in her thoughts. She should remember that he died a rapist, and that he took all the horrors he had committed with him into the grave (and they remain part of the truth about him). They do not stick to her.

"No, he is the one who has to answer for them to a higher judge," adds Mrs M, who has been listening attentively. She suddenly seems relieved. How could she have allowed her uncle to wander around like a ghost though every day of her life! She shakes her head. She doesn't want him in her presence anymore. Okay, she will go to the cemetery and say goodbye for good.

Lukas: Here my colleague brilliantly applied the method of the "imaginary dialogue"[11]. Experience shows that it is possible to hold

---

[11] First developed Berkeley, California by Joe Fabry, a close friend of Viktor E. Frankl.

a dialogue with a dead person. Almost everyone who has lost a loved one – or is far away – is able to converse with this person in spirit. The spiritual dimension easily transcends space and time. However, one rarely thinks of communicating with a person who is *not* loved. This, of course, is because one doesn't want to.

We know from logotherapy that conversing with a dead person can have a healing effect, especially if one of the two conversation partners has injured the other in some way. I myself have experienced surprisingly good examples of this type of dialogue. For example, in the case of women who regretted having an abortion years later. They can receive peace of mind from an imagined dialogue with their unborn child, in which they accept the child in a motherly way and apologise for shortening its life. Once, I advised a distraught mother, who had discovered the hanged body of her 19-year-old daughter and was constantly screaming, "How could my daughter have inflicted such suffering on me?" to have an imagined dialogue with her. After that, the mother was much more composed. She swore that her dead daughter had confided in her that "it wasn't her fault". I had to admit that the daughter was right: according to the medical report, she had suffered from severe depression – and it was not her intention but this illness that killed her.

This example shows how the sensitivity and insight of the living party is sharpened in these exceptional situations so that he or she is able to receive the words that the dead person might have spoken. In some mystical way these signals are almost always comforting.

Schönfeld: When we meet a few weeks later, Mrs M reports that she found her uncle's grave. It was in a rather inaccessible corner of the cemetery, where it was completely undisturbed. At first, she found it very difficult to recollect anything good about him. For decades, the good memories had been buried under the terrible event that was constantly in her mind. As soon as they came back to her, however, she was able to speak openly and honestly with her tormentor. Tears flowed down her cheeks, but they were no longer tears of anger. She saw him standing silently in front of her, his head lowered with guilt. She stood and contemplated this for a long time.

Back home, she thought at first that the trip had achieved nothing. But soon she noticed some significant changes. The stabbing thouhts that had plagued her every morning on waking had completely evaporated. Now she starts her day with more swing. At work, she has often received the appreciative comment: "You look so happy today!" Her colleagues feel comfortable around her. She confesses: "This has never happened before. All my life, I have retreated and protected myself to avoid being hurt again...now I can open up without fear." I'm happy for her. She is so glad to be rid of her ghastly memories.

Mrs M asks me how paedophilia comes about. Why men get so carried away that they commit such brutal acts. I explain to her that it involves both predisposition and bad conditioning. We all have acquired and/or inherited inclinations that provoke us. Some people are disposed to addiction or dependency. Some have a choleric temperament. Some are highly strung and inhibited. The important thing is to oppose bad inclinations and develop useful talents. I tell her about Frankl's analogy of the builder and the building material. Our heredity, our impressions, our physical characteristics and all socio-psychological influences are the building materials thrown at us by fate. *As a spiritual person*, we decide what to build with them: a prison or a hostel, a slum or a cathedral.

An inclination to paedophilia is a difficult burden. Looking at pornographic photos (which have proliferated like a plague on the internet) intensifies the pressure until the affected individuals throw aside all ethical considerations and act out their needs at the expense of children. We do not know whether Mrs M's uncle was a paedophile, that is, whether he was almost incapable of "normal" coitus. In any case, he could have sought professional help. Support is also offered by self-help groups, in which people overwhelmed by "abnormal" sexual desires unite and exchange strategies for prevention in order to avoid becoming "perpetrators". None of them can be absolved of their basic personal responsibility.

What is remarkable about the scene at the uncle's grave is that he did not defend himself (in Mrs M's imagined picture) and did not belittle what had happened. *He merely lowered his head and remained silent.* This can be credited to him: it was appropriate for him to stand before her in a posture of guilt. It is even more gratifying that Mrs M's resentment about her childhood has subsequently dissolved. Her soul is at peace, and the world around her enjoys her pleasant charisma.

Lukas: Mrs M originally contacted my colleague for help with her sleep disorder. It is questionable whether there is indeed a connection between these sleeping disorders and Mrs M's childhood trauma, as the patient suggests. I personally doubt it. My interpretation is that Mrs M also has a problematic tendency to brood. Despite the trauma, it is unusual that at 36 years of age she was still preoccupied with thoughts of what happened when she was 11. However, the fact that she is constantly preoccupied with thoughts about her uncle, despite her marriage, work, children, and rehabilitation from stroke, is probably not the cause of her sleeping problems. As in big things, so in small: Mrs M will also tend to brood over domestic problems, daily news, future plans, etc. – and when will she have the leisure to do so? When she goes to bed in the evening or wakes up at night.

This is incompatible with restful sleep. Restful sleep requires relaxation and letting go of the day's worries. Just as dogs have to be exercised regularly in order to "run themselves out", our brain needs to "run itself out" on a regular basis. Chasing dreams makes it sleepy. Keeping it, cognitively speaking, on a tight leash, will probably induce it to rebel from time to time.

My colleague skilfully defused her patient's constant negative thoughts about the past. Next, she will have to put an end to the brooding thoughts that keep her awake at night.

Schönfeld: It is time to treat the insomnia Mrs M mentioned at the beginning. She normally goes to bed at ten o'clock and it takes a long time for her to fall asleep. Around 2 am she wakes up again, and then she turns back and forth in bed until she has to get up early in the morning at about 6:30 am.

I tell her that Frankl's thesis was that the duration of sleep is not the most important thing. If one is deprived of enough sleep for several nights in a row, the body restores itself by entering into a deeper sleep. This may mean that someone who has slept only a few hours but deeply awakens more refreshed than someone who has slept for a long time lightly. Therefore, she should not worry about the number of hours of sleep she gets.

I also present her with an insight from studies on sleep. In an article in SZ online from 4 April 2018, it was shown that sleeping through the whole night is a myth. Peter Geisler from the Regensburg District Hospital found that sleeping people sometimes wake for a few seconds up to ten times an hour without realising it. In his view, this is a mechanism for survival in uncertain times, allowing people to check on a continual basis whether danger is approaching. These brief seconds of awakening, however, only tear us out of sleep when a bright light flashes, a noise thunders past, a baby screams or – when we are *overtaken by worries*.

So we need to know how to let go of worries. Worries and strange men have no place in her bed, I joke. Mrs M laughs. She should tie up all the worries, big and small, that she can think of in a bag in the evening before going to bed, and stick it in the freezer or the basement. She can promise herself that she will unwrap her worries again in the morning, but the night is a "worry-free zone", reserved for something more important!

I play around with a paradoxical thought: why waste the night with sleep at all? Sleep is boring! I ask her to describe the most beautiful place she has ever been in her life. Mrs M does not have to think for long: it was during a holiday on an island in the South Sea. There was amazing white sand, a row of palm trees, clear water. Excellent! This is the best place for her to fly away to in her imagination! Mrs M should close her outer eyes and open her inner eyes wide. She should see how the beautiful white sand glistens on the island's shore. She should let it slip through her fingers and feel how warm it is from the sun. Then she can listen to the gentle rumbling of the waves. The waves come and go, come and go, come and go...she can feel the gentle breeze blowing towards her from the waves. And when she looks up, she can see the palm leaves swaying in the whispering wind, back and forth, back and forth, back and forth... "Stop, I'm already asleep!" laughs Mrs M, fascinated. "Walk a little along the beach, maybe you'll find some shells," I suggest. "You could cover yourself with sand. Or you could stretch out in the shade of the palm trees. Or splash your feet in the sea...isn't that fun? Much nicer than a boring night of sleep! When you lie down in the evening, you should think: "Who wants to sleep? Let's go to the dream island!"

Two weeks later, I am curious to see how Mrs M has fared on her "island". It didn't always work, but she is much more relaxed and rested in the morning than she was before. Knowing that the duration of her sleep does not matter has helped her a lot. She no longer has to force herself to try to sleep. She has also discovered flowers and an exotic forest on her "island". Exploring it or swimming in the sea makes her tired, she says with a smile. Perhaps she is simply a person who does not need much sleep. When she lies relaxed in bed and "forgets to worry", but imagines a landscape instead, she feels completely restored and can jump out of bed in the morning full of energy. She is very grateful.

Lukas: To create a "dream land" for a patient requires a careful collection of personal preferences. Not every patient will respond to the idea of an island. In the case of Mrs M, however, this imaginative picture seems to have fulfilled its purpose, namely a successful "dereflection" (Frankl). You cannot order people *not to think* about something, such as critical problems or urgent tasks. Persistent, unwanted thoughts can only be stripped away by instructing them *what to think about instead* – something that provides them with calm, comforting feelings.

One might have explored whether Mrs M's love for horses was still latent in her. If so, an imaginary horse farm, full of magnificent animals with waving manes and funny raised tails, would also have made an ideal dream land. She could sit in the grass, leaning against the gate, breathing in the smell of the animals, watching the movement of their muscles, listening to the sound of hooves turning and turning in circles... Of course, this picture would not have been completely free of risk. This is because she had memories of a horse farm that were connected with her uncle.

Nevertheless, Mrs M is old enough to distinguish between innocent animals and guilty people. To me, it seems a pity that her love of riding and horse breeding has completely disappeared over the years. But she is still young. Who knows what the future holds for her?

Schönfeld: In parting, I tell Mrs M about a metaphor of life as a mosaic (Lukas). It contains both dark and light stones. Some are gemstones, like Mrs M's children, her friends, her husband. There are also precious stones that she has added by emerging bravely from the trauma she has suffered. In the middle of it all sits a jet-black stone. Does this stone deserve to be in the middle? Oh no, she says, she has long since placed it to one side. Admittedly, no stone can ever be removed from the mosaic once it is there (it cannot be deleted from the truth). But the empty spaces between the stones can be filled for as long as she lives. Mrs M is willing to select the most precious stones she can to complete her mosaic. She is struck by the idea that she can insert bright stones alongside the dark ones that have been added by fate. In the future, she will increase the bright contrast by not letting herself be shaken off balance by misfortunes, but responding to them with noblesse.

She has an idea. When she goes on outings with her family, she will collect colourful stones, small feathers and twigs. She will ask her husband to make her a photo frame with a thick border. In this frame, she will make a collage, a mosaic that will represent her life. She will be careful to choose what dominates in this picture – after all, she is the master builder. It is not the building material that will determine the shape of her collage, but her alone…

Mrs M leaves my practice with her head raised and a spring in her step.

Once again, I was able to witness that no trauma can break a person if the "will to meaning" wins out.

Dealing with the Pain of Grief

Lukas: It is no secret that we all have to die. But although we know this, we usually ignore this knowledge in how we live our lives. We think and act as if everything will go on forever, thinking only about the quality of our continued life. Few people dare to face openly the possible death of themselves and their loved ones, at least not without a compelling reason. This is why disastrous events and sudden deaths shake us up so much. They destroy the illusion of "eternal continuation" and force human beings to their knees. All tokens of power – possessions, fame, social status and prestige – are stripped away at the inexorable boundary that lies before us. It seems monstrous to us as soon as we have really grasped it, and this takes time...

Nevertheless, it would be good if we were able to face the topic of death while we are still alive (and if possible without being forced to by circumstance). This does not mean that it would be less hard when relatives or friends are taken away. The pain of grief is inevitable. We would, however, live less wrongly and less greedily and set our standards by a different measure: not by our imagined future, but by *our own identity.*

The neurologist Viktor E. Frankl drew attention to the fact that, unlike the tokens of power, our identity – defined as the sum of all qualities that characterise us and combine to form our ego – survives our death intact. Why is this? Think, for example, of a grandmother who has a warm and loving relationship with her grandchildren. What happens when she dies? It remains true that she *was* a warm, loving grandmother. Death can certainly terminate her existence, but it cannot change who she was and what she was like, it cannot retroactively turn her into a cruel and repulsive granny. It cannot touch the quality of a lived life; death has no power over historical truth. What has entered the truth has become true once and for all, and therefore our identity remains untouchable forever. This is true in every respect. Think of a miser who never gives anything away and only stores up money for himself. *This*, too, is stored in the permanency of truth as the personal identity of this individual.

Of course, one can say: *"Après moi, le déluge.* A century from now, no one will know who I was and what I was like..." That's true: on this earth everything will be forgotten. Despite all commemorative plaques and history books, in the end everything is extinguished. However, even what is forgotten does not disappear from the record of truth. And perhaps what is true somehow counts in a realm beyond this world? Frankl took the view that, in the end, everyone creates their own heaven or hell, depending on what is written about them in the record of truth.

If you follow this train of thought, the question of what really matters in life takes on a new aspect. There can be no value in hoarding possessions and luxuries, which one must relinquish sooner or later, at the point of death, if not before. There is also no lasting value in being honoured and admired by people whom one must leave behind sooner or later, again at death, if not before. What ultimately matters must be what lasts beyond death, and only *the truth about ourselves and how we lived* does this. Therefore, the only valid answer to the question is that what matters in life is to make oneself into a person with whose identity one can be satisfied in the deepest depths of one's soul.

From this perspective, the duration of a life is of little importance, but the values realised in a life are of great importance.

Schönfeld: A caller explains on the phone that she employs a carer to provide assistance to her elderly father. The family has become very fond of this carer. Right now, everyone in the family is very worried about her, because two months ago her son died. The carer is a bundle of misery. Although she performs her duties with her usual care, she is worryingly close to a breakdown. Could I schedule an appointment with her? This is how 58-year-old Mrs N arrives in my practice.

I can see that she wants to pull herself together, but soon she is crying bitterly. Little by little, the following story emerges.

Mrs N grew up in the suburbs of a big city and after leaving school, she worked in the catering industry. She became pregnant, married, and had a second child. Ten years later, shortly after the birth of her third child, Tom, her marriage broke down, and her husband left her. She struggled along for years as a hardworking single mother with her three children. She decided to move to another part of the country, because she believed that she would have better prospects there, but this proved not to be the case. So she continued to struggle. As soon as her two eldest children had grown up, they started families of their own and moved to a distant city. Mrs N found a small apartment in the countryside for herself and her youngest child; the apartment was cosy and affordable. Tom began an apprenticeship in a large bakery. He had a long commute by bus and train, but this did not bother him.

Mrs N was looking for a new field of professional activity and accepted an offer to retrain as a carer for elderly people. She liked to work with elderly and frail people. It suited her friendly and personable manner. An advantage was that this training lasted only one year, and Mrs N was able to finance it despite a shortage of money. She saw this as an opportunity for her future, so every day she walked an hour and a half each way to the training centre to save the cost of the bus.

This was the beginning of a good time in her life. There was a shortage of skilled workers in her field, so she immediately found a job in a mobile care station, and she performed her job every day with admirable engagement. Tom also successfully completed his apprenticeship and was taken on as an employee by the bakery. His salary was not large, but he had a profession he enjoyed that offered him opportunities for advancement. His mother was helping him to look for an apartment near his workplace. During this good time, Mrs N had managed to save some money, so she took her first holiday in a long time: five days in a thermal bath at a discounted price. What a rest! From there, she talked to her son every evening. On the third day, a Friday, Tom reported that he had stomach cramps. These were not bad, but they were painful enough that he stayed home from work. Surely he would recover by the end of the week. When asked, he answered that he did not want to see a doctor, because his pain was not that bad. Mrs N suggested some home remedies: he should drink chamomile tea, put a hot water bottle on his stomach and stay in bed. She would be back home in two days.

The next day, she couldn't reach Tom on his phone. She texted him several times, but received no reply. After half a day, she couldn't bear the worry any more. She talked on the phone with Tom's siblings and some of his work colleagues, but nobody knew anything about how he was doing. Finally, she asked Tom's neighbour, whom she knew, to ring Tom's doorbell and, if there was no answer, to enter Tom's apartment with the spare key to check on him. Soon after, the neighbour called her back: Tom was lying dead in the living room.

Mrs N suffered a nervous breakdown. The neighbour picked her up in his car.

Lukas: This is how it is with the terrible tragedies that one absolutely cannot understand, against which every human feeling revolts, that simply run counter to any sense of what is right and just. It cannot be – and yet it is. Never, never, never will you be able to make terms with it. Never, never, never will you be the same person you were before the tragedy. Something is irretrievably broken.

This is how it is with the treasures that one receives in the course of one's life, which seem as though they were contractual entitlements: they have their own radiance, their own greatness, their own existence in space and time, no more and no less. Appearances are deceptive. These things do not "belong" to us, they are not granted to us for all time, but only as temporary fiefdoms. Consider a jewelled necklace, 40 cm in length. It enhances and delights its wearer, even though it is not 50 cm or 60 cm or 70 cm long. Perhaps the wearer would like it to be longer, but she is unlikely to discard it because of its actual extent. The same thing applies to the treasures in our lives. Most of the time we would like them to be bigger, but the fact that *we have received them in their actual extent* is a wonderful gift!

Mrs N received a wonderful gift in her son, Tom. If she had not given birth to the boy, she would not have had to expend so much effort bringing him up. She could have afforded more things for herself, and above all, she would have no cause for grief now. Would that have been better? If one were to put this question to Mrs N, she

146

would certainly answer with a horrified denial. Of course not! The gift of Tom (in its actual extent) was worth the effort and the financial burden! Was it also worth the immense pain of grief? What would Mrs N choose, if she had a choice between no Tom and no grief or Tom – including the grief?

In my practice, I have often asked people who have had to mourn the death of a loved one an analagous question. None of them has ever chosen against the dead person. Each of them, after thorough reflection, has recognised the treasure of the person's presence in their lifes – *in its actual extent*, and has expressed sincere gratitude for it. A necklace 40 cm in length is worth much more than nothing. Likewise, to have a son for 20 years is worth infinitely more than having no son. What is irretrievably broken in Mrs N is neither her love for Tom nor her joy in his having been there. These things have a right to continue. As I said at the beginning, death destroys the illusion of "eternal continuation"...

Schönfeld: Two months have passed since the tragedy. Mrs N cries and sobs. I ask her to tell me about Tom and she tells me astonishingly positive things. With her two older children there are all sorts of difficulties: her eldest son is considering a divorce, her daughter unnecessarily put her job at risk and is now unemployed. Unlike them, Tom was diligent and reliable. He saved up money to pay for his driving test himself so that he wouldn't have to ask his mother for the money. He was a peaceful soul, and it was easy to get along with him. He had a cheerful disposition, he was helpful and popular with everyone. "With your description," I interject, "you are almost erecting a monument to him." She nods. Yes, she can't talk about Tom any other way, there was never any quarrel with him. If they disagreed, they could always work things out by talking. There was never any animosity about it. Her last phone call was also good. "Don't worry about me," were Tom's parting words to her as he lay at home with his stomach pain.

I pick up on this. Is not this a blessing in the midst of all the indescribable suffering? There were no harsh words spoken between them, and there is no unexpressed anger to darken her grief. Her pain has to do solely with the loss she has suffered. There are no missed opportunities for warmth or communication to add to her burden. I know of cases in which the death of a relative has occurred unexpectedly, and there was no opportunity to say the important words, "Forgive me." In these cases, there was no possibility of reconciliation, and this exacerbated the loss like a corrosive acid. She is "fortunate in her misfortune", in that during her son's lifetime she was able to develop and maintain such a harmonious relationship with him.

Mrs N agrees in tears. She wants to be strong, she forces herself to be functional, but she is overwhelmed by pain all the time. She would have cried for any of her children, no matter what they were doing and how they lived. Of course, she loves all her children very much, but with Tom she had something extra special. They had lived together for almost all of his life, and they got along perfectly. She had always had to keep an eye on the two older children, who occasionally went off the rails, but for Tom she had nothing but pride. He was the most precious thing in her world.

Lukas: There is nothing wrong with a little retrospective glorification of a son. This is appropriate for the grieving heart of a mother. We can never judge the past with complete objectivity, and we are always biased by our current point of view.

Incidentally, this is the dilemma faced by all historians. If, for example, one knows how a battle will end, it is hard not to think that the competing armies should have foreseen the outcome and acted with more wisdom. At the time of the battle, however, the situation was completely different. This is also the case for testimonies given to the police or in court. An assessment made with the benefit of hindsight rarely coincides with the assumptions and plans that are made before the event.

Experiments from psychological and biological memory research prove that the past is always viewed through tinted lenses. In the case of patients of psychotherapeutic practices, these lenses are often coloured darkly. The patients judge their childhoods or their past lives to be more dreary and oppressive than they were in reality. But there are also the colourful lenses of the "good old times" which are unfortunately in the past – and often did not go quite as smoothly as the memory suggests.

However, even if this phenomenon is taken into account, Mrs N is right to "put up a monument" to her deceased son. More accurately expressed, *Tom has put up a remarkable monument to himself.* We have already seen that a person's identity does not disappear from the record of historical truth, but rests secure in it. And what is written there under the name of "Tom", what belongs to him forever, beyond the grave, is altogether lovable and pleasant. It is the identity of a person who has been hardworking, peaceable, cheerful, reliable, considerate, etc. from an early age. A person who grew up without a father and with a sometimes overwhelmed mother, who had to cope with moving to a different part of the country, and with restricted financial circumstances, and who nevertheless, despite puberty and post-puberty, had no problems leaving the nest. A person who has proven himself in his strenuous work without complaint or shirking and who has earned the goodwill of his fellow employees. A person who was able to resolve family conflicts constructively and was a friend and support to his ageing mother. One can only congratulate her unreservedly! What a successful life! And his death takes not the slightest bit of this away from her.

We should remember this while we are still alive: "Every act is its own monument!"(Frankl). What kind of monument do *we* carve into our being?

Schönfeld: I point out to Mrs N that there is a connection between her great grief and her great love. Each implies the other. There are people for whom no one cries when they are dead. There are people whose relatives breathe a sigh of relief when they die. And there are anonymous deaths that do not affect anyone at all. In her case, however, there was a deep love, a "love that lives on in her grief". She likes what Frankl says about this. I tell her that during his internment in a concentration camp during World War II, Prof. Frankl did not know whether his young wife, whom he had only recently married, was still alive. This did not prevent him from entering into an inner dialogue with her. He later wrote that he would not have communicated with her any less intimately if he had known at the time that she was dead...[12]

Treading carefully, I pursue the following train of thought: Mrs N is not a poor woman. She is "rich". Every one of her tears expresses her wealth. She has been enriched by a happy period of time with her son. She has a great treasure in the treasure chest of her life. Poor people are the ones who do not possess such treasures, the ones who *never have to grieve because they have never loved*. Mrs N answers that if her present pain has to be as enormous as the good that came before, then it will last for a long time. Perhaps it will. However, she should not defend herself against her grief, but welcome it, because it is the sign and seal of an indissoluble connection between her and her deceased child.

Because of work, Mrs N can't come back to me until three weeks later. This time she smiles a little, but she confesses that she still sometimes bursts into tears all of a sudden. Her friends suggest that she should move out, because there is so much in her apartment that reminds her of Tom, but she doesn't want to. She likes her apartment and she likes to remember her son. She says that as he wanted to

---

[12] Frankl, V.E., *Psychotherapy and Existentialism: Selected Papers on Logotherapy.* New York: Simon & Schuster, 1967, p. 109.

move into his own apartment, she would have been just as alone in the apartment if he had lived. In tribute to the inner wealth we have been talking about, she has bought a bucket of paint, put on a one of Tom's old t-shirts (a symbol of his closeness to her) and repainted his old room so that she can live in it herself. I encourage her in this. This is a step towards psychic "resurrection". Tom would be pleased with her!

We talk about suffering. It spares no one. Many people want to keep it at bay. They think, "out of sight, out of mind", and are prescribed sedatives and sleeping pills to numb their pain. But the suffering cannot be kept away, it wells up again all the time. Mrs N is more daring: she confronts her pain and carries it. She has photos of her son on her breakfast table – and she can stand it. How wonderful! In this way, he remains "with her".

I sum it up: Tom is a treasure in her life, he is close to her, and he is doubly secure: first in the eternal truth, with his attractive identity, and secondly in her heart and in her unbroken motherly love. There is no strife and discord to cloud her memories of him. Instead, her mourning can take on a new form: a *profound feeling of gratitude.* Relinquishing the claim to eternal continuation, she has every reason to thank fate for having been given a son like Tom.

Lukas: When human scientists, inspired by the war atrocities of the 20th century, spent years studying post-traumatic stress disorders and how to treat them, they came across the exceptional talent of "resilience". Just as people can be incredibly brutal, more satanic than in any nightmare, they can also be more noble and angelic than one could imagine. The heights to which people are able to ascend include major sacrifices accepted for the sake of other people, or the capacity to transform unavoidable suffering into a personal achievement. Frankl related many touching examples that he experienced in the concentration camps. The spiritual capacity of human beings is truly staggering...

The clinical term resilience now denotes an ability to process dramatic experiences with heroic acceptance and to shape the nature of one's survival in a triumphant fashion. Some people are immune to the shadows cast by dreams. They go through terrible things, they buckle, they burn with pain, but then they rise again and set about shaping the rest of their lives with a skill that even makes fruitful use of their horrifying experiences. Specialists ask what gives them the power to do so. Is it their trust in God? Is it a motivating vision? Is it their power of defiance against all-powerful fate? We don't know. So far, only *one* common feature has been identified: they can all give themselves to the "meaning of the moment" (Frankl) without being held back by the events that they have experienced.

Momentous events always place us on a threshold between two stages of life. The earlier stage of life has come to some kind of end, because one of its "continuations" has been cut off. In Mrs N's case, this is the living contact with her son. The new stage of life must first be entered and examined. If it is only defined by the emptiness left behind by what has been cut off, we will shudder back from it. This can mean that *in the present* we remain standing on the threshold for a long time, because of all the misery behind and all the discomfort ahead.

One thing, however, must be made clear: *the present is the only time we have at our disposal.* If, blinded by anger, resentment, or wistfulness about the past, we fail to make full use of the meaning of the present, it becomes past, and we are confronted with the future – a future in which, in addition to the existing sorrow, we will have reason to lament our failures in the present that has just passed. And everything flows inexorably into the unerasable truth. To put it bluntly, this means that *what you bungle today is bungled forever – and you will regret it tomorrow.*

Studies of traumatised war veterans have shown that their psychological wounds can be healed by coaching young people in a sports club or volunteering. Studies of accident victims found that the people who made the greatest and most rapid progress with rehabilitation were those who did not allow themselves to be overwhelmed by anger and upset about the causes of the accident, but focused on adapting and coping with their present circumstances. These things by no means exclude grieving over what has happened – instead the grief is integrated into a new approach: *because* life is valued more highly, and nothing can be taken for granted as "self-evident", the present is shaped more carefully. Something like this is happening with Mrs N. She is less willing to miss out on fulfilling the "meaning of the moment". In addition to coping with her full work schedule, she redecorates her late son's bedroom. My colleague cleverly supports this growing resilience in her patient, and this protects her from falling into reactive depression.

Schönfeld: In a later session, I talk to Mrs N about the possibility of joining a support group for bereaved parents. Self-help groups can provide much comfort. They reinforce the knowledge that one is not alone in one's suffering, but lives amongst fellow sufferers whose circumstances are similarly difficult. It is well-known that pain is easier to bear if it is shared. Individual sufferers also know that other people who have also suffered can understand them better than anyone else. People who have not experienced similar things cannot really understand them. Comforting words from non-sufferers always feel empty, which is a difficulty for all who try to intervene in a crisis. In self-help groups, it is possible to meet with people who know exactly what it's like…

In support groups for bereaved parents, the principle is that parents have to pull themselves out of total despair *for the sake of their dead children*. To despair is to burden their dead children with the responsibility of having triggered a catastrophe for their parents. The children, however, should be allowed to remain what they have always been: a source of joy for their parents. Whether they lived for two months or twenty years, their existence should still be and remain a cause for joy! Mrs N is immediately convinced by this argument. Her Tom was far too good to be responsible for his mother's breakdown. And was he a cause for joy? A hundred times yes!

Mrs N is shaken into alertness. Tom wouldn't like it at all, she says, if he saw her crying all the time. He always appreciated the things she had bravely accomplished in her life. Well, he can still do that now, I suggest.

The idea of what Tom would think of something has become relevant again. It is almost the time of an annual fair that Mrs N habitually attended with Tom. There was a certain stall where they used to enjoy snacking on pretzels and roasted almonds and bought balloons. They went there every year and always had a good time. Should Mrs N go there this year? Won't the bustle of the fair around her be particularly hurtful, as she is so deeply in mourning? And what will her friends think if they see her enjoying herself at a busy fair only six months after the death of her son? So is it better to stay at home? She hesitates.

We think about what Tom would advise if he were sitting here with us. This is hard to guess, says Mrs N. She thinks about it for a long time, but finally makes up her mind. Tom wouldn't like her to be hiding at home. All her life, she has been a strong woman who has overcome with tenacity all the blows of fate that have come her way and the difficulties that they caused, and this always impressed Tom. Nothing could get the best of his "strong Mum". If he could talk to us today, he would want his "strong Mum" back. A mother who couldn't be held back, and stood up bravely to the challenges of life. So she has no doubt that Tom would be happy for her to go to the fair.

What would be better for her: to remain contentedly at home – there is nothing wrong with that either! – or to go to the fair? Suddenly, Mrs N decides she will go to the fair and head straight for the stall that sells pretzels and roasted almonds. She will get herself some, whether or not her cheeks are running with tears. She will also buy some balloons and say to Tom: "I'm letting them fly up to you, my son!" Then she will return home, and even if her heart is wrung with pain, she will be able to say to Tom: "Look, I want to be brave...I am so glad I had you...for your sake I'm plodding on so that you can be proud of your Mum... See how in every minute, in every tear, in every difficulty I face, my love for you lives on."

Lukas: Our life has many stages. We are not finished beings, and our life's work always remains fragile and unfinished. We can only make an *honest attempt* to seek, find, and actualise the possible meaning in any situation. There are no guarantees. We can neither be certain that what we believe to be meaningful is actually meaningful, nor that we will succeed in actualising what we have recognised as meaningful. Failure is an inevitable part of being human.

But perhaps that "honest effort" is enough, regardless of its outcome. Perhaps the small fragments that we eventually bring into being are enough. There are "unfinished works" in all areas of art, some of which are amongst the most beautiful. And, in art, what matters is not the extent of a work, but what it has to offer us.

Sometimes it is necessary to correct the usual measures of value, based on prestige, wealth or education. The short life of the good baker's assistant Tom was a *miniature work of art*. In remaining steadfast in the endurance of her grief, his mother is adding a valuable detail to the work of art that is her own life. It would be great if we learned the following from Mrs N's story as we think about the topic of death:

1. Everything we have is granted as a temporary fiefdom, and nothing on earth belongs to us. The only thing that truly belongs to us is the truth about ourselves.

2. There is no need for monuments, because every person carves his or her own monument by choosing how to live.

155

3. The work of art that is a human life is evaluated according to higher standards than what is socially desirable.

Learning these truths would lift us spiritually by several degrees of development.

Schönfeld: One month later, Mrs N visits me again. She has regularly attended meetings of the support group for bereaved parents. She tells me about a memorial she attended with this group in the cemetery, which was very touching, but also very upsetting. However, she takes this as a sign and seal of the indissolubly good connection between her and Tom.

Then she talks about her work. In one of the families to whom she provides care, there is young mother whose newborn child is terminally ill. She has empathy for this situation. A 92-year-old lady for whom she provided care had to go to the hospital. There Mrs N visited her privately, and the elderly lady was surprised and pleased. Clearly, Mrs N is fully integrated into the present. The "meaning of the moment" also draws her to her two adult children, about whom she is worried. Both are in difficult situations, and Mrs N wants to be there for them.

I see that Mrs N's perspective has widened to include other people's suffering. This helps her immensely. Her great suffering, which had confined her like an iron cage, has broken, releasing her will to live. What a positive healing process! Her grief for her son will never disappear, and nor should it, because her motherly love will continue forever. Grief will become a faithful companion in Mrs N's life – and so will gratitude for her Tom.

A famous quote from Frankl says: "Suffering makes people clairvoyant and the world transparent."[13] I believe that Mrs N has won

---

[13] Viktor E. Frankl, *Logotherapie und Existenzanalyse*, Belz, Weinheim und Basel, 2010, p. 136.

this clairvoyance, which is why I can release her from counselling with confidence.

Brave Odette

Schönfeld: Viktor E. Frankl's logotherapy is conceptually very challenging. His works are all based on a deep philosophical framework. His psychological interventions, his concept of the human being and his theory of human motivation have all been thoroughly worked out using this framework as a guide. Although his therapeutic methods appear on the surface to come easily and spontaneously, they always have a well-founded theoretical basis. Students of my courses in Frankl's original logotherapy here in Bamberg realise that you can't get far with Frankl without considerable effort.

This is sometimes made into an accusation against logotherapy. It is said to be a cognitively difficult system understandable only to educated people – it is simply too highbrow.

The opposite is true. What sets Frankl apart is that he has made the basic outline of human existence clear. He has emphasised being human, and put this at the centre – as the basis both for a psychologically stable life and for therapeutic treatment. What makes us human is what he called the spiritual (noetic) dimension. This distinguishes us from the cleverest animal not only quantitatively, but qualitatively.

This is the core of every human being, regardless of intellectual ability and education, and this also applies to people for whom an intellectually demanding approach is inaccessible.

For example, I myself have had good experiences using logo-therapy with children.[14] A student of mine, Johanna Sandau from Bochum, Germany, goes even further, and uses logotherapy with disabled people. She is an artist by profession, and also an art thera-pist, a practitioner of psychotherapy and a logotherapist. Her freelan-ce work often takes her to residential care homes for people with mental disabilities.

"Mental disability" is a term commonly used for cognitive im-pairment and various physical, psychological and intellectual limita-tions. People who suffer from such disabilities are often unable to participate in normal everyday life on their own. However, these disabilities do not apply to what logotherapy calls the spiritual di-mension. According to Frankl, the "spiritual dimension" is the essen-tially human component of every human being. It is human dignity, irrespective of health or illness. "Mental disability" describes a con-dition of cerebral dysfunction which has an effect on thought proces-ses and behaviour. According to logotherapy, however, people who suffer from a mental disability, do not suffer from any spiritual disa-bility.

Lukas: Frankl was aware that the term "spiritual" – despite the long Western tradition of the concept of spirit – is ambiguous and easily misunderstood. In the German language, "geistig", the word for spi-ritual, is often equated with "rational". In English, "spiritual" is in-terpreted as "religious". What Frankl meant by the term "spiritual", however, is the specific quality that makes us human, and, as my colleague says, gives us humans our personal dignity. This quality is essential to our existence, whether we are young or old, clever or stupid, wide awake or sleepy. Because of this semantic difficulty,

---

[14] Elisabeth Lukas and Heidi Schönfeld, *Meaning-Centred Psychotherapy*, Elisabeth-Lukas-Archive, Bamberg, 2019. "Florian, Fritz and Jürgen", pp. 173ff.

Frankl introduced the Greek-derived term "noetic" in his writings, a term which is familiar to only a small number of experts. It doesn't seem important to me for the technical vocabulary to be widely used. But what is important (and seems to be becoming increasingly important in our time) is *unconditional respect for every person* – regardless of race, culture, gender, age or state of health, and regardless of any prejudices that may arise from a conception of their external or internal state. *This respect is founded on a recognition of their humanity.* What really unites us in this world is simply our being human – in Frankl's words it is the noetic dimension. As one can rely on this on a small scale, for example in the therapeutic process, it would be advisable to hope for it on a large scale, because without it we would be nothing more than a pack of werewolves snapping at one another's throats.

Schönfeld: Johanna Sandau can relate many successful examples of her work with disabled people. With her generous permission, I would like to report one of the most touching examples here.

This story is about Odette. She is a young woman, 27 years of age, who is negotiating her way between supervised care and an independent life. She was raised in extremely difficult family circumstances, and she was born with fetal alcohol syndrome. Odette and her two equally neglected siblings were admitted to welfare institutions soon after birth, because their alcoholic parents were unable to care properly for their children. Odette has a mild intelligence disorder and can read and write to some extent. She attended a special needs school. After ten years of school, she moved on to vocational training in a workshop for people with disabilities. There she spent two years training in various fields of activity. She did best in woodworking, so she stayed with this for a long time.

Odette understands that she is different from other people. She has a small head and a small nose that immediately stand out. More serious, however, is her developmental disorder. She has the mental level of an eight-year-old child; her practical skills are a bit more advanced. Various attempts to live on her own or even enter the labour market have failed. In the meantime, she lives in a shared residence, where each resident has a self-contained apartment, but is still connected to a larger community with professional staff.

As a result of her mother's alcohol consumption during pregnancy, her brain experienced prenatal damage, the effects of which are twofold. Odette has both a cognitive disorder and a psychological instability leading to strong emotional fluctuations, which often sink her into depression.

Odette receives various kinds of independence training from her carer. One element of this is to practice how she can withdraw small amounts of money from her bank account. She is not able to operate an ATM. For cases like hers, the bank has set up a special counter staffed by employees, where people with disabilities can withdraw money.

When the carer went with Odette to the Bank for the first time to practice the process at the counter, Odette stopped in front of the entrance to the Bank and suffered a panic attack. She became stiff with fear, trembled all over, and was unable to move a step further towards the entrance. She cried, hyperventilated, and was so distraught that the carer thought she might faint. The carer had no choice but to take Odette back home.

A few days later, Odette met Johanna Sandau, whom she already knew from her art therapy sessions. She told her excitedly about her terrible experience. The two sat down together, and a conversation began.

Odette described her great fear, how she had stood stiffly in front of the bank, how she could not get any further, how she had almost fallen down and how hard her heart was beating. She described the symptoms of her panic attack in simple sentences, and ended by saying that she would never go to a bank again.

Johanna Sandau listened and then asked what would happen if she walked into the bank. Odette immediately refused. No, she would never do that, she was afraid and had nothing but fear and she would never go there again. But Johanna Sandau was persistent and asked again what would happen if Odette dared to enter the building.

The Bank would collapse, said Odette without hesitation. And it would be her fault. Everyone would look at her in shock. It would be her fault because everything would go wrong. Then she wouldn't get any money. Perhaps people would laugh at her. But worst of all would be that the building would collapse and she would be to blame.

This is how Odette expressed her anxious thoughts – but she added: "I know this is all nonsense. But I can't help it. I think about it. I see it happen. I can't go in there."

Johanna Sandau questioned her further, asking how she knew all this. Odette immediately replied, "There's a devil on my shoulder, he tells me."

Lukas: If we were dealing with a person with no developmental disability, we would be worried at this point. Is this not beyond the scope of an anxiety disorder? Are we not dealing here with a touch of psychotic delusion? Do we have to resort to sedatives? However, because we know that Odette has the mental capacity of a child and, as a result, speaks a child-like visual language, we can assess her fear-induced imaginations as a neurotic overreaction. Perhaps she has seen films of collapsing buildings and associated them somehow with the word "bank". Or perhaps she has listened to fairy tales in which a devil has made similar threats. It is a rule in therapy that you should never rush in with the "heavy artillery", but always try more innocuous methods at first.

Schönfeld: With great therapeutic skill, Johanna Sandau immediately reduces the fearsome devil to a harmless little monster by saying

161

to Odette with a smile: "I know what you can do next time. When the little monster is squatting on your shoulder again, you just say to him: 'Hey, you up there, if we go in now, then the ceiling will fall down on our heads with a big crash! But let it be so that everything turns to rubble and nothing is left at all. The whole building will be lying around us on the ground and all the people will stare at us stupidly. Watch out for Odette's superpowers, little monster! Only I can do this,' you will explain, 'no one else can manage it! Everyone will be amazed!'"

Odette is surprised. She looks questioningly for a moment – and then bursts into laughter.

The whole encounter lasts less than ten minutes. Johanna Sandau takes her leave, saying: "You'll see, this will be great fun! You will be Odette the Bank Destroyer, and all banks will be afraid of you. The little monster will be allowed to watch you destroy the bank three times in a row, every time you take out some money."

A few days later, the two run into each other again. Odette, radiant all over, runs towards Johanna Sandau with a laugh, and reports: "I did it yesterday! I withdrew money from the bank!"

There is no more talk of fear.

Lukas: Readers will of course recognise that Johanna Sandau used the method of paradoxical intention. The "devil" has been driven out of a fearful soul by means of humour and exaggeration. We do not always need to know how unnecessary panic manages to embed itself into the psyche. One can speculate, but in the end one can never know much about it. However, there is *one* thing that is almost always involved, namely a feeling of inferiority. Odette is clearly not "disabled enough" not to understand that other people have an advantage over her. Others are able to do things that she cannot; and, as we have said, this is not entirely invisible to her. The possibility of being laughed at may also have played a role in her anxiety. It was very clever of Johanna Sandau to enhance Odette's powers in her paradoxal narrative. *She* has superpowers, others must be afraid of *her*... What fun it is to be strong and brave, even if only in the imagination...

Odette does not realise that it is more than a fantasy. As the spiritual person she *actually is*, she does possess superpowers for coping meaningfully with the disability she *has*. Her mental limitations must indeed capitulate to her spiritual being – for spiritually she is completely healthy, an unbroken, precious human being. If we believed otherwise, we would have chosen a different profession.

Schönfeld: Odette, the young woman with fetal alcohol syndrome, chased away her unnecessary fears with laughter and opened up a new area of life for herself. All anxiety sufferers could learn from her – and all therapists could learn from Johanna Sandau, who translates Frankl's sophisticated therapeutic methods into simple language, using them accurately and effectively to help people with disabilities.

Thus, "highbrow" logotherapy heals by allowing what is genuinely human to prevail over psychological disorders, and even over intellectual limitations.

Frankl on "True Love"

(Elisabeth Lukas interviewed by Heidi Schönfeld)

Schönfeld: In my practice, it strikes me how differently the phenomenon of love is often understood and interpreted. There seems to be no universally valid view of love.

Lukas: I have written more than once about the chapter "The Meaning of Love" in Viktor Frankl's great work, *The Doctor and the Soul*. You are right. This text is enormously touching, but it is difficult to reconcile with how love is lived and thought about in our time.

Schönfeld: Here is one thing I noticed about this chapter. Frankl conceived/wrote it before he was in the concentration camp, in the early 40's (and later extended it). You can sense this, because the reality of his love and relationship at that time shines through. I wonder what would he write today, if he could see how much sexuality and relationships and love have changed? He would probably not write something completely different – but he would discuss current phenomena. That would be fascinating.

Frankl concludes – independently of morals – on purely logical grounds that true love is based on faithfulness and duration, which is very insightful. But today, lives like this are rather the exception. In earlier times, marriages were sometimes formal and remained intact on the outside until death – but they were certainly not all happy. Two people often had to stay together for financial reasons, mainly because women have only recently been able to lead independent "single" lives.

What about true love: A and B have found each other, they both fall in love sincerely and in the whole depth of their being, i.e. they see and love one another as they can be at their best. All is well.

But years go by, and humans necessarily change – not only for the better, but also for the worse. One always has to make decisions – and can also make bad ones. Suppose B opts more and more for material success, rises in the world and receives advances from prettier, younger people – and thinks, why not? So B gets involved in extramarital affairs.

What has happened to the love? Has B's original love evaporated? It was supposed to last forever, but has B grown out of it?

What about A? Does A's love remain steadfast? B has indeed changed a long way from the best version that A saw. Perhaps B's behaviour has become unbearable for A. Does A now revise his love because B has become another person? Then the love was not permanent.

There are many A's and B's. Sometimes they break up badly, sometimes they sort themselves out, usually they separate. I can count many variations on this theme amongst my acquaintances. It is also not true that they never really loved one another, that would be an incorrect allegation. One cannot simply reckon retrospectively like this: Those who remain together love truly; those who break up love only in an emotional or physical sense, but without spiritual depth.

Why does love end when it was once completely real and sincere and true, and saw people as they were "intended by God" (Dostoevsky)?

Or does one have to think like this: Is it a new question every day for lovers whether they love one another; the existential encounter must always be freshly renewed. This would mean that a love that is no longer renewed dies.

Or does Frankl paint with beautiful words an ideal of which humans should be worthy – but it is like a distant star which guides us, but which we cannot reach?

Or does one really love, stop loving, and after a good holiday/ book/seminar/couple's therapy, find the way back to love. Then love might progress in waves.

There is a second thing in this chapter that I find very difficult. In a footnote in the subsection "Psychosexual maturity" he writes, "Just as little or as rarely as the average person is capable of true love, just as little or as rarely does he reach the highest stage of development in his love life." But the lofty goal must exist.

This is very daringly formulated, and it seems to disparage "the average person". I think that every "average person" can love genuinely – if not neurotically disturbed or egocentric or something. Otherwise, Frankl's whole concept is not true – A life form that hardly anyone attains cannot be deeply appropriate for every human being. It sounds rather elitist when Frankl describes average people so badly.

You, Dr. Lukas, knew him well personally. Did he really think this way? Love as an act of self-transcendence – if this what makes people the most human – how can it be beyond most "average people"?

Lukas: My dear colleague, you have asked me a lot of questions at once. They refer to Frankl's book *The Doctor and the Soul*, in which he described "true love" between two people in a very touching way, distinguishing it from "merely" erotic and sexual relationships. This true love is lasting – and Frankl lived it out in a marriage lasting more than 50 years.

I admit, however, that if we look at the partnerships around today, the question arises whether, with his demanding concept of love, he sketched out an ideal of a more aspirational than actually achievable nature. As you say, he himself admitted in the book that the average person would rarely reach the highest level of development in love. Since Frankl otherwise held in high regard the healthy human understanding and feeling of the "man or woman in the street", in other words the average citizen, this assessment seems a little pessimistic. Is the gap between Frankl's love-ideal and reality really so enormous, and did Frankl know this?

It is certainly a pity that we can no longer ask him. However, the texts reissued in his later years make it clear that Frankl was by no means dispossessed of his "ideal" by modern partnership practices. He was the one who studied the uniquely human element, the human spirit, and thought through it with the utmost consistency. And spirituality includes a *pure sense of valuation* of one person by another, without any desire for possession.

Perhaps a metaphor can help us here. When a hen walks along a path, everything is checked for its usefulness, in this case, its edibility. If a sparking diamond were laid before her feet, she would ignore it because of its uselessness. The hen has no access to the value of "beauty", particularly "beauty in itself". However, a spiritual being like a human does have such access. A human being can kneel down and be captivated by the beauty of the diamond. Naturally the "hen" is also present in every individual. The diamond is not only beautiful, it is also useful, because one can make money from it. So the person greedily reaches for the diamond.

A researcher who wanted to bring out the spiritual spark in a human being would have to separate the person from the plumage of the "inner hen". He or she would have to filter out this amazing human potential to be able to enjoy pure beauty from the muddle of covetousness, commercialism, and egotistical calculation so that it could be known at all. Indeed, it is only a spark, and if it is not blown into life, it might fade away to such a dull glow that it is easily overlooked. Then the theory of being human would be reduced to the "level of the hen".

It is probably similar with Frank's concept of love. He defines love as *the deepest sense of the value of the loved one*. The animalistic side of us, of course, wants something different. It wants advantages, affection, sex. It wants something from the beloved. Expects something. It is wonderful if this all adds up to peaceful unity, and the sense of value continues to fill sober everyday life with its light. But diamonds are not edible. To apply this analogy: If the partner's advantages and affections are withdrawn, if he or she does not fulfil expectations or, yes, perhaps even behaves abominably, which can happen, then the sense of value is reduced.

In particular, if people do not (or no longer) bring to realisation the unique value that is latent within them, their partners will find it increasingly difficult to see it. But with the decline of the sense of value, "true love" disappears, even though by nature it is supposed to last, *because the value of the originally beloved person is also supposed to last.* A diamond remains a diamond. But who admires the beauty of a diamond encrusted with dirt?

This is how it is: the human spirit is a spark in a sea of ashes. That is why the human capacity for true and unselfish love is rare. Let us nevertheless be grateful for this spark: it lifts us over the heads of the "hens" into the heavens, nosedives included. And let us be grateful that someone like Viktor E. Frankl has so persistently made us aware of this precious spark in us. Who is he a dreamer, an idealist? I do not think so. Rather, I believe that he pointed us to a meta-reality that encompasses our reality, and at the same time opens up the prospect of a better humanity on the distant horizon of the future, in which the spark – we hope – may shine more brightly than today.

Making Up and Making Good[15]

(Heidi Schönfeld)

The chapter "Dealing with feelings of guilt" tells the story of little Eva, whose death caused her carer so much grief. In contrast to the largely unjustified feelings of guilt described in this case study, we often encounter cases of actual guilt in psychotherapeutic practice, and the pressing question arises of how we can address this guilt therapeutically. How can guilty people best conduct their lives under the shadow of their misdeeds?

In logotherapy, we always emphasise the inner dignity of the person, even a person who is ill. We often focus on the potential for humour (cf. the case study about Odette). This is because humour is specific to human beings. No dog laughs, no cat tells a joke.

Also specific to human beings is the dark side of being human: the fact that they can become guilty. This also distinguishes us from a dog and a cat. A fox that bites into a goose's neck is not guilty. The phenomenon of guilt is reserved for us humans. It is a fundamental pattern, a basic possibility of human existence, the logical consequence of our freedom and responsibility.

Guilt has such great importance in Frankl's work that together with suffering and death it makes up part of the so-called tragic triad. This tragic triad affects all human beings without exception. None of us can go through life without being guilty, just as none of us can be spared grief and death.

Not least for this reason, we often have to work in our therapeutic practices with people who have become guilty - and probably even more often with people who are tormented by feelings of guilt.

---

[15] Abridged version of a talk given at the International Congress of Logotherapy in Moscow in 2018.

In religion, guilt normally has something to do with God. If I betray someone, I become guilty towards that person, but at the same time I become guilty towards God, because I am breaking his commandments. All guilt separates me from God and requires his forgiveness. In a religious context, one speaks of sin.

Logotherapy will not and must not say anything about these religious connections. As a branch of medical psychology, it has to do with worldly connections and not otherworldly ones. Thus, when we talk about guilt in logotherapy, it is always a concept referring purely to the inner world.

We find a general concept of guilt in everyday speech. One often says, "I'm guilty, it was my mistake," where the "mistake" is some small error or unintentional oversight. Or causal connections are made, for example: "The weather is to blame for my bad mood." None of these trivialisations do justice to the topic of human guilt.

When we talk about human guilt in logotherapy, it presupposes two things:

1. A person must have had freedom of action, for example, an opportunity to prevent a disaster. There must have been a free choice.

2. A person must have known (to some extent) what it would have been meaningful to do in a particular situation. In other words, the person must have had the ability to recognise the meaning of the situation.

Example 1. A man in a wheelchair sits at the beach and watches a child struggling and drowning in the waves. If the child drowns, it is not the man's fault, because he is paralysed and unable to get out of his wheelchair. He does not have the free choice to rush to the child's aid. He may be in desperation at having to look on helplessly, but he need not and should not reproach himself.

Example 2. A patient complains, "If I hadn't been on this trip with my friends, I would have been at home when my husband fell. Then he would not have had to lie helplessly on the stairs for hours until someone found him." Well, no one can see the future. No one can know in advance that a disaster will happen. The patient had no meaningful reason to cancel her trip. There is no guilt here.

Guilt requires both freedom of will and understanding of meaning. Notice that *the question of meaning does not arise if free will is not present* [16] (it does not arise for stones, plants, animals, babies, people in comas...) *It manifests itself for us only within the context of our human free will.* For the paralysed man, the question simply does not arise whether it would be meaningful to jump up and rescue the drowning child from the waves. Another question may be relevant for him, for example whether he could summon nearby people on the beach by shouting. He has the freedom and power to shout. In the above examples, where there is free choice, it must be preceded by an awareness of meaning in order for guilt to arise (as a result of non-compliance with that awareness of meaning). But where there is awareness of meaning, the option to follow it *always exists*. This is why, according to Frankl, freedom of will is *prior* to the will to meaning.[17] Only a free being such as a human can go on to be a be-

---

[16] Of course, human beings can also inquire into the meaning of situations about which they have no freedom of choice, such as the meaning of something or even of *everything* that exists. Frankl said laconically: "It is meaningless to ask about the meaning of existence, because existence is prior to meaning. For the existence of meaning is assumed when we question the meaning of existence. Existence is, so to speak, the wall we are backed up against whenever we question it." Viktor E. Frankl, *The Doctor and the Soul*, New York, Random House, 1986, p. 196.

[17] Frankl built his logotherapy on three axioms: 1. The freedom of the will, 2. The will to meaning, and 3. The meaning of life.

ing who seeks meaning, not vice versa. If a search for meaning is already in motion, freedom of will has long been available.

I repeat: guilt is only possible if someone knew in the first place exactly what should have been done (or not done) and could meaningfully have done it (or not done it) – and did *not* act accordingly. Something that was worth actualising, and that could have been actualised, was neglected. What was done was contrary to one's own conscience.

We need to define all of this carefully, so as to distinguish a genuine sense of guilt from the inappropriate feelings of guilt that we so often encounter in psychotherapeutic practice.

Inappropriate feelings of guilt can have many causes. They may be the result of psychosis. If a person's perception of reality is distorted, it may lead to all sorts of exaggerated guilt feelings. In particular, endogenous depression often causes irrational feelings of guilt which have no correspondence to reality. If a severely depressed mother feels guilty because she cannot prepare breakfast for her children, this inability is a result of her illness, and not because she does not love her children. The guilt feelings experienced by depressed people can inflate into surreal ideas of condemnation and nihilistic depersonalisation, known as "wandering melancholy".

Excessive feelings of guilt are also often a burdensome symptom of obsessive-compulsive disorders. If a person feels guilty for touching a table top on which other people have to eat with hands that are only 99.9% clean, or for staring at odd door numbers, which might be unlucky for the residents behind them, then these feelings of guilt are symptoms of illness. Naturally, we must not react as if this were genuine guilt. That would be a terrible mistake.

There are also insecure, melancholy, unselfish people who occasionally feel guilty about something for they have no actual responsibility. One must listen to them very carefully and distinguish the unnecessary guilt with the help of the criteria of freedom of will and awareness of meaning. One must free these people from their inappropriate feelings of guilt, which is often not easy.

How do we deal with unjustified feelings of guilt therapeutically? Without a specific diagnosis, it is impossible to create a therapy plan. A psychotic illness requires a carefully chosen and balanced medication, which can largely eliminate distorted ideas. In cases of endogenous depression, we need to identify the guilt feelings as symptoms of the illness and advise patients to ignore them using dereflection. In cases of obsessive-compulsive disorder, inappropriate feelings of guilt should be parodied using paradoxical intention, as we have repeatedly illustrated. When insecure people mistakenly declare themselves to be guilty, one must point out their mistake. "If I hadn't allowed my child to play at the neighbours' house, he wouldn't have fallen from the tree." – As we said, no one can see the future, no one can prevent every accident. "Enough suffering – away with feelings of guilt," is the motto.

Fact: Unjustified, partly irrational feelings of guilt can be traced back either to a mistake or to an illness. And we must do everything we can to eliminate them therapeutically.

What do we do, however, when a patient has genuine, existential guilt?

First of all, Frankl wrote at length about whether it can be meaningful to grieve or repent about what cannot be changed. What does this achieve, when one can no longer do anything about it? Is this a hopeless effort? Frankl came to the following conclusion:

"Thus there is revealed in man's emotions a deep wisdom superior to all reason, which in fact runs counter to the gospel of rationalistic utility. Consider, for instance, the affects of grief and repentance. From the utilitarian point of view both necessarily appear to be meaningless. To mourn for anything irrevocably lost must seem useless and foolish from the point of view of 'sound common sense', and this holds also for repenting an irredeemable wrong.

But for the inner biography of a man, grief and repentance do have meaning. Grieving for a person whom we have loved and lost in a sense continues his life, and repentance permits the culprit to rise again freed of guilt."[18]

This is an exciting and thought-provoking statement. From the utilitarian point of view, all grief is a completely useless waste of strength, it cannot bring a dead person back. And yet love somehow allows the loved one to live again in the grief and it does not allow itself to be disturbed by death. How precious!

At the same time, Frankl explained his thoughts on guilt. Does it matter whether or not I regret something I did? What has happened has happened, why should I feel bad about it, since this helps no one? Frankl leaves behind this feeble utilitarian way of thinking; life doesn't work like this. Rather: *"...the repentance of a guilty person somehow enables that person to rise again, free of guilt."*

If I could experience again today the situation in which I became guilty, and if I can say that today I would behave differently and not incur this guilt, then today I have become a different person to the person I was then. Something fundamental has changed! Something new has arisen!

More precisely: whenever I cause someone else to suffer, I simultaneously lose my lack of guilt, my integrity. The German language makes this very clear: to say "I'm sorry" one says, "es tut *mir* Leid," it causes suffering to *me*, I have also done something to myself. Repentance doesn't eliminate this, but it produces reconciliation, it "pays off" the suffering, as Frankl says, making use of a banking concept. Repentance allows one to pay off the guilt in one's account. This does not make it unreal, but it settles the debt. In this respect, repentance makes me into a new person, it prevents me from causing

---

[18] Viktor E. Frankl, *The Doctor and the Soul*, New York, Random House, 1986, p. 108.

yet another person to suffer in this way, and somehow metaphysically pays off my debt of guilt.

Let us return to the question of what we, as logotherapists, have to offer people who are aware that they have "existential", that is, genuine guilt.

To make the boundaries clear, I must first say what we *cannot* offer. We can offer no psychological absolution. This sounds rather banal, but behind it lies an ongoing professional dispute that never seems to end and has lasted an entire century. "I am only so aggressive because I was raised so carelessly." "I steal because I was never given enough toys as a child." "I only do what everybody else does."

All his life, Frankl took his stand against this sort of psychological absolution and said, plainly and clearly: "Anyone who takes guilt away from human beings (i.e. denies it), also takes away their dignity." This plunges us back into the contended determinism of "I couldn't do anything else, because…" – Frankl says no to this.

So what can we offer guilty people? A worthy answer to existential guilt is called "reparation". This word has a triple meaning: 1. To make good an injury to another person 2. To bring light to another person in the darkness 3. To become a new person by means of repentance. All of these are forms of reparation. The first has the highest priority. For example, if you have offended someone, you ask for forgiveness. If you have stolen something, you give it back. This is the best way. If this is no longer possible, however, for example because the whereabouts of the injured party is unknown or all contact is blocked – in other words, if the best way is unavailable – then reparation is still possible. One engages where one would not otherwise have engaged. One practices "active penance" and "all the good things that would not have happened without me testify to me" (Lukas).

The third way is for the difficult situations in life when the first two ways are both closed off. It may be that someone is very ill, has a severe disability, is in prison or lying on their deathbed, and there is nothing in the world that they can make good again. Frankl said exactly this to the death-row intimate Aaron Mitchell in San Quentin State Prison: he still had the last and "highest" possibility open to him, by climbing – internally – through his repentance to a higher level and dying as a better person than the one he had lived as. Guilt then becomes an impetus for inner change, and in extreme cases this is possible even on one's deathbed.

Fortunately, in psychotherapeutic practice we can mainly work with the first and second way.

However, it becomes difficult when justified and unjustified feelings of guilt are combined. I would like to illustrate this with a case study in which a small amount of genuine guilt was combined with unjustified guilt feelings that lasted for decades.

In the case of an 85-year-old doctor, who had been coming to me for therapy for some time, a problem came to light by chance towards the end of our sessions. He reported that he did not know whether he was responsible for his father's death. The following story emerged:

After a routine examination, a small malignant tumour had been removed from his father. After that, the father fell into depression because the fear of cancer nagged at him day and night. He no longer took care of himself, he no longer worked, and he repeatedly said, "I will kill myself before I die of cancer." Medically, there was no actual reason for concern, and the family looked after him patiently, but they were helpless in the face of his repeated suicide threats.

One day, on September 30th, the father came to his son's surgery in the evening, formally dressed, and invited him to join him for a walk and dinner in a local restaurant. The son, however, was buried in his accounts, for it was the end of the quarter, and there was a huge amount of administrative work in his newly opened practice. So he answered his father: "I don't want to today, I still have so many accounts to settle." The father looked sad and left. That night he killed himself.

Is the son guilty?

What is certain is that the son could not have prevented the suicide. This decision was and remains the responsibility of the father (if the father was suffering from a severe depression, his personal responsibility for the suicide would be even less). I asked my patient if the two criteria of a clear awareness of meaning and freedom of will were satisfied.

A clear awareness of meaning? Certainly not. If he had foreseen the danger, he would certainly have found time for his father. But how could he have known that on that September 30th he was seeing his father alive for the last time?

Freedom of will? Well, his quarterly accounts were pressing...

I wanted to convey to the man that there was no personal guilt on his part. Nevertheless, a silent doubt hung in the air. "I let my father go away sad" – he had freely chosen that. This could not be eliminated from the man's story. For this, there could be no appeal to excuses such as "I would not have done that if I had known that he would die so soon". To let his father leave in sadness – on any evening – was not a great choice, regardless of whether they would see one other again or not. *In this respect there had been an awareness of meaning!*

We accepted a small debt of guilt for my patient. Then I searched with him for a larger context for this small guilt. Yes, he had also had many enjoyable and fruitful conversations with his father. Unfortunately, the antidepressants the father was taking did not bring him any relief. Against the background of the father's entire life, his life-long achievements came to light: he had been a kind and reliable father until his illness, he had provided his sons with a good education – for which he had had to work a lot of overtime – and many other things.

The conclusion from our deliberations was that my patient should find a place where he would feel close to his dead father. There he should focus on his memories of his father and speak to him – and then *listen* for a kind of "response" from the father in his heart.

The memory exercise was a great success. My patient later told me that he had hung a photo of his father over his desk, in which he could be seen sitting in the garden as a young man with his wife and children. To *this* father he could confide everything that had eaten away at him since that terrible day of September 30th. He apologised to his father, and asked for his forgiveness. And he offered him sincere thanks for all the good things that he had experienced from him throughout his life.

Since then, the doctor's sense of guilt had eased. He had expressed regret to his father for letting him go away sad and he had admitted that he had not understood the drama of the hour. What remained was the memory of their good times together and his thankfulness for it. The nagging doubt was gone.

Sometimes it can be the other way around: something bad has been done to someone, and the culprit has died before it could be spoken about.

I had one such patient. Again, it came up as a throwaway remark which was not to be ignored. He said, "I hate my father. I have never experienced anything positive about him." My enquiries revealed the following:

The man's father had had serious alcohol problems and was apparently a good-for-nothing. He had betrayed the man's mother in every way, leaving her soon after the son's birth, and he never took any interest in the child. The son could not remember a single pleasant encounter with him. All he knew was that his father had soon been taken in by another woman and had died of severe alcoholism a few years later.

The son, who had grown up in the meantime, was left with nothing but contempt. He loved his mother, and he had simply never had a father – that was all! He had not gone to his father's funeral and he had never visited his grave.

But I could not let my patient go away with hatred and contempt in his heart: people who keep such things in their hearts carry a heavy burden on their shoulders.

We talked for a while about his father, and tried to understand a little why he had fallen into alcoholism. There had only been a few good years with his mother, but at least there had been some. On reflection, it became ever clearer that his unwillingness to look after his son was the result of a great helplessness and incapacity on his part, because he was not in control of his own life and he was in no position to take care of his son. This was in no way to justify him! But it made it possible to understand him a little.

I asked if it wouldn't be good if the son could "talk" about all of this with his father, to speak out his accusations against his father for once, all of his overlooked desires as a child, so that he could finally say: "You didn't do a good job as a father, but I don't hold it against you anymore."

My patient actually did exactly this. For the first time in his life, he went to his father's grave and told him about all the hurt he had suffered as a child. This big grown-up man had never cried so much as he did at his father's grave. There in the cemetery, a great compassion welled up in the poor man's heart and washed away all the grudges and reproaches.

He went on his way and was free.

All of these examples demonstrate that asking for forgiveness and forgiving cannot be prevented by death.

The Top Ten Frequently Asked Questions.

(Elisabeth Lukas)

A doctor friend of mine searched on social media for the most frequently asked questions about psychology today. The extensive random sample revealed ten main topics in the following order:

1. Depression
2. Work stress
3. Family disagreements
4. Experiences of failure
5. Educational problems

6. Addiction
7. Becoming old and weak
8. Decision-making conflicts
9. Competitive pressure
10. Letting go.

The above-mentioned topics clearly reflect that the people of our time suffer from great difficulties and concerns. For this reason, I have compiled some brief information for anyone who needs advice.

Depression

From a professional point of view, there is a lot of confusion about the topic of depression. Sometimes uneasiness, dejection or shyness is all-too quickly labelled as depression. Melancholic character traits or introverted behaviour are carelessly attributed to depression. It is quite normal not to be happy every day or to get down if you are in an uncomfortable or exasperating situation. Life alternates between laughter and tears, and reasons for laughter are in the minority (and therefore all the more precious). The fact that antidepressents are requested and prescribed just because there are genuine reasons for crying is nonsense. Just as our body is provided with the ability to heal itself, our psyche is well equipped to cope with stress. If this task is delegated to medication at every opportunity, the psyche forgets how to do so.

One should only speak of depression in a clinical sense when the psyche is unable to heal itself – that is, when there is an *illness*. Depressive illnesses can be rooted in many very different aspects of human existence. It is the task of the specialist to carefully determine what type of depression is at work in a patient, and to resort to anti-depressants only in the case of a diagnosed *unipolar or bipolar disorder*. Simply expressed, these disorders are irregularities in the release of neurotransmitters at the synapses of the nerve pathways, and this leads to periods of unipolar depression occurring at times that have no connection with the patient's external circumstances. If there are manic periods in between, one speaks of a bipolar disorder. Whether there are triggers for these periods of "derailment" is a matter of opinion. Relatives and acquaintances of the sufferer tend to blame the recurrence of the illness on any unpleasant events that may have occurred, but there is no evidence for this connection. Statistics show that it is likely to be a hereditary illness that can skip generations, but is prevalent within certain families.

It is different with so-called reactive depression, for which there is not just a trigger, but a genuine cause for grief. But note that this is no natural grieving process. Grieving is right and good if, for example, you have lost a loved one, or if you have been afflicted by a severe blow of fate. What is loved and precious should not be forgotten, but kept in the heart, and this is the purpose of sorrow. It preserves a connection to what has been lost and an awareness of its value. Unfortunately, however, grief can develop into a sort of mental rigidity. The griever retreats like a hermit crab into its shell and says: "If I can't have the one thing that was dear to me and that I lost, then I don't want anything! I won't be there for anyone anymore! I'm not interested in anything in the world anymore!" Individuals who have built all their happiness on this one thing that has now been taken away from them are especially at risk of this kind of reactive depression. Single-minded valuations and overvaluations come at a cost. For example, if a woman thinks, "I can't live without my lover," she has laid foundations that are at risk of collapse should her loved one ever leave her. Or if a man thinks, "My business means everything to me," he comes up against a mental abyss if his business ever has to be sold.

Antidepressants are of course of no benefit to people who have developed reactive depression. What they need is insight and reassurance. For example, the insight that everything we cherish is only on loan for a certain period of time. And the reassurance that *even after it is lost* it is a happy circumstance that it was part of our life for a time. As soon as gratitude is added to grief, the soul breathes a sigh of relief. If the insight that no earthly thing is to be overvalued is also grasped, some stability is restored.

There is a third form of clinical depression, namely the *noogenic depressions* identified by Viktor E. Frankl. They are reactive depressions in which the mental judgement, everything (= my beloved) *or* nothing, has developed into the summary dismissal, everything *is* nothing. The word noogenic[19] indicates that the clinical concept refers not primarily to a mental slump, but to an ingrained mental frustration, a chronic absence of values in life, in which the sufferer no longer knows where to find meaning. In most cases, there are no adverse blows of fate involved. On the contrary, noogenic disorders are often considered a product of civilisation, because they spread most prolifically in the most favourable life circumstances. Individuals who are affected feel bored, uninspired, wile away their days without joy, and wonder why they are alive at all. Nothing arouses their interest, nothing spurs them into physical, emotional or mental activity. A heavy indifference hardens them to the world's problems.

---

[19] The Greek word nous means spirit.

Antidepressants are useless in these cases. The only way out of this crisis is to reactivate one's sensitivity to values and fundamentally correct one's philosophy of life. Frankl's logotherapy provides the arguments that are needed to tear such patients out of their lethargy and heal their frustrations by leading them to a search for meaning and, if necessary, by challenging their existential orientation.

Work pressure

If two acquaintances run into each other on the street and ask how the other is doing, then the answer is likely to indicate that things are not bad, but there is a lot of pressure at work. It is clearly considered good form to emphasise work pressure. In reality, this is not a good thing, and not only from the perspective of health. Persistent work stress makes reflection and planning impossible in daily life, and this has drastic consequences.

According to many surveys, most people in our society want more rest and relaxation. This is a legitimate wish, but strange: just as many people are very active in their time off work, undertaking activities from shopping trips to long car journeys and overseas travel, from internet surfing to long hours of film watching, all-night partying, and numerous social events. The busyness people complain about is often rooted in their own hearts and in a lifestyle led by distraction rather than inward contemplation. Genuine inner calm and silence, without constant inundations from the outside world and the distracting temptations of a smartphone or tablet, has become hardly bearable. The busy people of our hectic times are not used to it. They would have to sit quietly in a corner for a while and meditate. Or stroll along a riverbank looking at the water. Or look up at the night sky and let themselves be awed by the twinkling stars. All this has become particularly foreign to city dwellers.

It is easy to explain why the absence of pauses for rest and reflection in daily life leads to drastic consequences. The body is not adapted to continual focus and multitasking, and will do what it needs to do to enforce a break. The brain decreases its capacity for concentration and signals fatigue. The psyche cries out to be numbed and switched off, which is often achieved with the help of alcohol or other substances.

Meanwhile, the spiritual being loses contact with the inner voice that judges *what is essential and what is not*. It spins in the hamster wheel without reflecting on whether or not it is meaningful to continue in its established routines. Bestselling author Stephen Covey perfectly expressed this stage with the metaphor of sharpening a saw. One tortures oneself by endlessly cutting down trees with a uselessly blunt saw, in order to avoid "wasting time sharpening it..."

In other words, work stress (if it occurs) *needs* to be compensated for outside of working hours. In Western cultures, there is a strong urge for creative activity, which is not bad in and of itself, because creative power is a sign and attribute of humanity. Trying to do too much, however, achieves nothing. It is also a sign and attribute of humanity to be able to appreciate and enjoy beautiful and unique experiences. Mastering the art of squeezing in precious mini-adventures (hiking in the forest, daydreaming in a scented bath, listening to beautiful music, reading good stories, having stimulating conversations, etc.) between intensive periods of work provides immunity to the negative effects of work pressure. Occasionally adding a completely quiet break will forestall any possibility of burnout.

Perhaps we should consider the origin of the word "stress". Hans Selye, who first used the term in a medical context, described it as the spice of life. For him, stress was a motivator to develop innovative solutions to incident problems and to develop one's experience. Later, the term "stress" developed increasingly negative associations, and was reduced to a sense of burden. Selye's distinction between beneficial "eustress" and pathological "distress" has not prevailed in public usage. The two are miles apart. As Frankl put it, eustress signifies a healthy "noodynamic tension between the ideal and the actual", that exists when one dedicates oneself enthusiastically to a chosen task. Distress, in contrast, relates to the tension of feeling unable to cope with a task that is imposed from outside. While eustress is characterised by affirmation and conviction, distress is driven by an – imagined or justified – fear of failure.

Fundamentally, however, *people cannot be expected to do something of which they are not capable.* They should not expect it of themselves, they should not allow any authority to impose it on them, and they should certainly not harbour the delusion that it is absolutely necessary. I am not blind to unavoidable constraints that force some people into a tight corner, or to tricky situations where one has no idea how to proceed. Nevertheless, this rule remains valid: *life does not require unreasonable things from us*; only reasonable things are expected. So, what should we do in a crisis? Here silence is more necessary than ever! We need to protect ourselves from all interference and look inside. We need to listen to what our inner voice is telling us. We need to weigh up our real task: what we are meaningfully "meant" to do (in accordance with our capacities)[20]. When we have recognised what this is, we can affirm it, no matter how difficult it is. By being aware that we are *in charge of our own actions*, we are freed from being defined by others. It is possible that other people expect something or other from us, but this should not be allowed to lead us astray. If we agree with them, we will accept the mission assigned to us. If we do not agree, we will insist on an alternative. It is appropriate for us to do our best, but this should be *of our own accord*, in harmony with the meaning we have perceived for ourselves.

Of course, if we are subjected to violence, our hand may be forced. But even the most controlling bosses have learned that their

---

[20] "Meaning is what is meant", as the Americans say!

subordinates achieve less when they are forced to act contrary to their inner convictions. The same happens when we act contrary to our own inner volition. If we are saying "yes" externally and "no" internally to an act, we perform it badly. This has nothing to do with stress, but with our own mental ambivalence. If, on the other hand, we say "yes" both internally *and* externally to an act, it is easy to perform it, no matter how stressful it is. In summary, therefore:

Doing what is meaningful does us no harm, even if it involves enormous effort. And doing what is not meaningful is unpalatable, even if it is easy.

Family disagreements

Modern societies are progressing (at a snail's pace) towards equal rights for women. Although this development is extremely welcome, it does not only bring advantages. Many women are torn between work and family, between career and motherhood. The scrabble for compromises becomes a hair-raising adventure for parents and a game of chance for their growing children, for whom every failure of their parents' search for compromise leaves scars. Politically, few solutions exist. Although quotas can be introduced to facilitate women's entry into male-dominated management roles, and childcare provision can be improved, a mother who is present is – at least for toddlers – worth much more than childcare. I don't mean to suggest that we should revert to outdated family patterns. I only want to assert that *children are worth making sacrifices for*, and that some of their parents' wishes should be put aside to give children the secure and warm environment that they need in their early years for successful development. Even getting a pet brings obligations. How much more does the birth of a child call for responsibility on the part of parents.

Family disagreements often have to do with a lack of willingness to compromise. In functioning communities, not everyone can get their own way. It's like an orchestra: the violinist can't just fiddle away mindlessly, the trumpeter can't always blast out loud notes, the bass player can't just pack up his instrument and leave. For the performance to succeed, all the musicians must cooperate to the best of their knowledge and ability. It is no different with family cohesion. What unites them and gives them strength is a common will to contribute constructively where their own talents are needed, and to withdraw gracefully when others are active. Just as an orchestra submits to the control of a conductor, family members do well to submit to a kind of "higher directive" that instructs them to treat each other with respect, to be tolerant, to refrain from aggression and to make peace in situations of conflict. If more families allowed themselves to be guided by this directive, there would be considerably less of the aggression in schools which currently causes so many difficulties for teachers.

There are three aspects of this worth looking at in more detail:

1. The first aspect relates to the *meaningfulness* or *non-meaningfulness of a sacrifice.* Children, as we have said, are worth making sacrifices for. If their mothers have enough time for them, if their fathers are present and provide a good role model, they have won the lottery. In general, it is noble to make charitable sacrifices. Many people in helping, caring and other professions invest more effort into their daily tasks than would be required by their job descriptions. Before we diagnose them with a helper syndrome, we should show them our respect, because no welfare state could function without them. Like family members who take on much responsibility and are always serving their family, they cannot be thanked enough.

However, mindfulness is required in such service. The driver of voluntary sacrifice should be spiritual love and not psychic weakness. If someone submits to the wishes of fellow human beings out of not daring to say no, this is not praiseworthy at all. If someone makes others dependent out of a desire for superiority, this is reprehensible. Likewise, if someone spoils family members and children in order to buy their affirmation and affection, this is nothing but a lousy trick. Meaningless sacrifices do no one any good and quickly degenerate into pathological dependency. Ultimately, people who sacrifice themselves meaninglessly make themselves ill, and people who are the recipients of unnecessary sacrifices are constrained in their autonomy.

For this reason, it is advisable to link willingness to sacrifice with mindfulness and to preserve the right to set boundaries in close relationships.

2. The second aspect focuses on the phenomena of *tolerance and intolerance.* These phenomena have been well researched in psychology. Intolerant individuals have an aversion to compromise, tend to look for allies, and exaggerate the "evil" of the villains against whom they fight, or humiliate and lecture those they think are villains. The star pianist Lang Lang once gave a gala concert in a Salzburg school. As he was practising for it in the morning, a window had been left open, and a lady from the neighbourhood promptly complained to the head of the school. She was completely beside herself, because some idiot had been plonking on the piano for hours, it was beyond endurance... When the audience called for repeated encores in the evening, Lang Lang told this story with a smile.

On inspection, this situation includes all the aspects we have just mentioned. The exaggeration ("completely beside herself"), the negative judgement ("some idiot"), the attempt to get the head of the school on her side and finally not having the goodwill to allow the school to invite a musician from time to time.

Intolerance divides up families with impassable lines. Each member of the family takes a side, and even attempts to draw in children for support. What the "enemy side" does is scrutinised with unfiltered criticism and even demonised. The suffering caused by the "enemy side" is rubbed in everyone's faces. One becomes increasingly entangled in imagined injuries that have nothing to do with reality. Sometimes a separation becomes inevitable. The only thing that can prevent this is sensitive communication *from the beginning*, not only to establish everyone's position, but to listen and try to understand one another better. This conversation should be conducted without resorting to allies, exaggerations and attempts at humiliation.

3. The third noteworthy aspect is *forgiveness instead of holding grudges*. First, let's make a small diversion. Achievement is widely regarded as a seal of approval. Children are encouraged to do well at school, and company bosses maintain this expectation with their employees. But what is the measure of human achievement? One might say it is *the conditions under which it is provided*. To speak plainly, the more difficult the conditions under which a person can show kindness, bravery or growth, the greater the achievement. If, for example, an ex-criminal stays clean and does honest work after being released from prison, then this is a terrific achievement! Hardly anything is as difficult as leaving behind a criminal past and beginning a respectable life.

If one interprets "achievement" in this way, the act of forgiveness is also a huge achievement. Hardly anything is as difficult as forgiving people who have done you harm. Everything in our being resists it, and yet forgiveness is a particularly powerful medicine, because it cuts through endless chains of suffering. The guilty party, freed from hatred, can have a fresh start. In the absence of hatred, it is also easier to make amends. And the forgiver shakes off the heavy baggage that comes from hating and bearing a grudge.

No community can do without the medicine of forgiveness, and particularly not an intimate group like the family. For whether we like it or not, we constantly tread on one another's toes. Human ignorance causes us to hurt one another. This is not an excuse – and unfortunately sometimes the injury is even done on purpose! It is merely a consequence of our psycho-social inadequacy. Only a generous willingness to forgive can compensate for this weakness.

Experiences of failure

The topic of forgiveness leads seamlessly into the topic of dealing with guilt and failure. As nothing can be erased from our life history, regret clings to us from every failure and error. Experience shows that people react to it very differently. Psychotherapy practices are full of people who harbour feelings of inferiority, tear themselves to pieces with endless self-reproach, and constantly complain that there is no possibility of happiness because of what has happened in their lives. Others try to pull the wool over other people's eyes, vehemently denying any guilt of their own and believing that the fault is always with other people. Both of these are questionable coping mechanisms

People who wallow in self-recrimination are of no use to themselves and others, and compound their failures even more. Instead of learning from their mistakes so as to avoid making them again, and instead of reducing the damage caused, they waste their resources on unfruitful self-accusation. Those, on the other hand, who are unwilling to admit their mistakes, deceive themselves. Not wanting to believe something may be a sign that deep down you know it to be true! Displacement is no solution. The best way to cope with one's own failure is to take the following three steps:

First, carefully examine whether this failure could really have been prevented. If not, all guilt can be discarded. You have had bad luck, but at least you are not to blame. If you are to blame, picture an imaginary old-fashioned pair of scales with two bowls and place all the failure in one of the two bowls.

Second, place everything that has been done successfully and capably in the other bowl. Perhaps the two bowls are roughly in balance. Even if they are not, this provides a broader view and prevents fixation on the negative side.

Third, take immediate steps to rebalance the scales by adding weight to the positive side. Direct reparation is not always possible. Some mistakes can no longer be ironed out. This should not discourage us, however: we can still balance the scales with small gestures of helpfulness, friendship, solidarity, and so on. The number of possible good works waiting for us is endless. If something has been botched, you can create something new and positive. If you have acted carelessly, you can remind yourself and others to be careful. If emotions have done damage, mastering them can impress others. Every corner of the world that we have made darker, – and which has been permanently closed to us – can be counterbalanced by shining a ray of light *into another corner*.

I have described the act of forgiveness as a huge achievement. The brilliant counterpart to this is for a guilty person to become someone better.

Educational problems

Errors of education belong to the category of errors that cannot be made good later. Thus, it is a good idea to avoid serious mistakes from the outset. Children are generally quite robust. They recover quickly from dramatic events and adapt well to external change. Refugee children, for example, are masters of integration. But what they need as an elixir of life is a picture of a secure world and a re-spectful self-image and concept of humanity. If these are not present, there are problems

On the picture of a secure world:
Early in life, a child discovers that he or she is an ego confronted with an outside world. In the first instance, this outside world is rep-resented by a single reference person, normally the mother. Children understand that the outside world provides them with food, comfort, support and tenderness. If they feel hungry, a spoon approaches; if they cry, a hand comes near to caress them. A picture emerges of a world that is benevolent and completely in order. As the child gets older, this picture fades into the background, and the child grows into the real world, where hopes alternate with disappointments and injus-tices emerge amongst what is right and fair. But in the background of thought and feeling, the secure world continues to exist as a trans-cendent and all-encompassing overworld and this strengthens basic trust. In contrast, children who have never experienced this sense of security are afflicted with a fundamental lack of trust that constantly undermines their healthy development. They can grow into basic trust in maturity, but this is a long process.

On the respectful self-image and concept of humanity:
In interactions with children, one sends unspoken messages that are easily imprinted on their learning brain. In particular, their self-awareness is shaped by how they are judged by their parents and other authority figures. How their parents talk to each other or talk about other people is carefully registered by their little ears (and souls). What the adults say is pieced together like a puzzle and ulti-mately builds up a self-image and concept of humanity. The most important message you can give to your child is: "You are a valuable person."

The message goes on. What it says is roughly as follows: "You are a valuable person, whether you are healthy or ill, whether you get good or bad grades at school, whether you have been obedient or disobedient – unconditionally!" Once you have sent this message, you can also reprimand children when they get on your nerves, react strongly when you are annoyed, ignore them when you are exhausted, and commit any number of other educational mistakes – children will not take it badly. Parents are also only human! As long as children know that they are valued, they are protected by an aura of inviolability.

There is more. In a climate of appreciation, they are also inclined to classify their teachers, their comrades, and their friends as valuable people, and thus to refrain from aggressive attacks in cases of dispute. One does not hit out at something that is valued. One does not want to destroy it. The same rule applies not only in families and stepfamilies, but also in politics at the highest level: *To reap peace, you must sow respect.*

We might ask what will be most important for the coming generation. Futurologists predict that it will no longer be the general knowledge that they have stored in their heads. We now have many super-intelligent "assistants" who will inform us at the touch of a button about anything that we don't already know. Other skills, in contrast, will be essential. Experts predict that *social skills* such as empathy, ethical sensibility and peaceability will be the most important. Unfortunately, school timetables are only very gradually taking this insight into account. The urgent recommendation to all educators and parents is therefore to worry less about whether young people are high achievers or get a good job quickly than about *whether they show respect for one another and their fellow human beings. They will do so unconditionally* (that is, regardless of gender, ethnicity, culture or religion), if they feel themselves to be unconditionally valued by their educators.

Addiction

Addiction is an ancient scourge of humanity. It is easy to fall into, and wretchedly slow to climb out of. It is by no means true that people do not fight against their addictions. Humans are the freest beings on earth, born free and not as slaves, and every enslavement offends human dignity. Nevertheless, the fact that millions of intelligent and educated persons fall prey to alcoholism, for example, can only be explained by the fact that physiological, psychological and social risks undermine their stability.

Physiological risks include genetic predisposition and feedback processes in the central nervous system, which produce euphoria when alcohol or drugs are consumed, and excruciating dysphoria when they are withdrawn. Those who cannot (or will not) endure long term dysphoria must get more of the addictive substance to escape it – at least in the short term. A prison wall builds up around the individual.

Psychological risks include the classic seducer away from meaning: fear. A person may be inhibited by nature, but able to entertain others marvellously under the influence of alcohol. A person may feel weak but develop a sense of iron strength under the influence of drugs. The nagging fear says: "You are not able to handle the demands of life, but you can prevail with the help of your stimulant!" Unfortunately, this victory is fleeting, and the need grows ever stronger.

Social risks include a lack of education and the social sanctioning of addictive substances. Wine, sparkling wine, beer and spirits are commonly consumed, especially on festive occasions. Smoking is a way to express one's individuality. Sugary and fatty treats are the most common gifts. Addiction to digital devices is whitewashed by the cry for more and more digitalisation.

Of course, all of this does no harm in moderate doses. But that's the sticking point. When people fall into addiction, they can no longer control the dose, and it gets bigger and bigger – until the individual breaks down.

It is therefore wise to abstain from time to time, to test for oneself whether the spiritual brakes are still in order. I know a man who abstained from alcohol for two months. He stocked up on provisions and had himself rowed by a ferryman to a practically uninhabited island with instructions to pick him up after the two months had passed. This was a radical step, but he succeeded in freeing himself from his growing addiction, which had already reached a dangerous stage. This method will not be the right one for everyone, but the idea behind it is sound. A change of location, getting some distance from one's usual surroundings, makes it easier to wriggle out of addiction. Silence and solitude enable one to take stock and think about how best to spend one's future life. All self-regeneration requires a strong "what for": *What should one change for?* Perhaps for love. For the sake of a loved one. For the sake of a task you want to accomplish. In order to enjoy a good figure and clarity of thought. Only the motivation of loving something can overrule the fear and lead one back to a meaningful existence – through the hell of withdrawal if necessary. And depending on the addictive substance in question, withdrawal can be extremely gruesome. Nevertheless, there is no greater triumph than triumphing over oneself!

Experienced addiction therapists suggest that the "what for" should be constantly kept in mind, using physical memory jogs. A photo of the children, attached to a bottle of spirits, might cause their father to withdraw his hand. A slender dress on a kitchen hook might prevent an overweight mother from opening the fridge. Frankl was convinced that humans have an intrinsic "defiance of the spirit", on which they can rely even if body and psyche are pulling them in the wrong direction. And there are many heroes who have proved that

Frankl was right. No one has to bow before the all-devouring moloch of addiction.

Becoming old and weak

Everyone needs to reckon up what has happened in their life, particularly from the onset of middle age. One reaches an age where the idealistic exuberance of youth has faded and the sobering insight sets in that time is fleeting and everything is fragile and ephemeral. A typical midlife crisis involves the anxious question of whether one is just getting old and weak. In fact, no one knows what the future will bring (which is perhaps a blessing). On the other hand, everything that is already in one's own past *can* be evaluated, specifically with regard to whether it has largely fulfilled its meaning. People have worked hard for things, they have received training, established contacts, taken on all sorts of work, set up a home, suffered setbacks and losses and picked themselves up again. It is good when someone is able to be satisfied with all of this! When one is able to say, "Yes, it wasn't always easy, but my life was worth living". Such a person can contemplate what is to come with serenity. Because everything that person has is protected in the following philosophical sense. Everything in the past is safe and protected from decay in the stronghold of truth; nothing that has been lived can be erased from its record. The past only appears to fade. In reality, it is the possibilities of the future that waste and ebb away with increasing age, until they dry up completely with our death. Our past, however, survives our death and remains – whether known or not – forever in history.

But what about when people are not satisfied with the outcomes of their lives thus far? Well, then there is all the more urgency to forestall the wasting of the future by actualising the best and most glorious possibilities of the present and stowing them in the safe shelter of the past. What can be renewed, seized, mastered, appeased? What undertakings should no longer be put off? What dreams should finally be realised? *Time is precious*, and the more conscious one becomes of this fact, the more carefully one will use it. Perhaps it is time to stop striving for material things and return to existential values such as helpfulness, cameraderie, friendship, musical appreciation, and so on. After all, *truth does not discriminate*. The evidence of our past and present being also encompasses jealousy, malaise or constant annoyance. And who wants to enter eternity with the attributes of a curmudgeon?

Let us not fear old age. It may bring wrinkles, weaknesses and disabilities, but it is full of illuminating possibilities until the end. Let us use every solitary hour not to complain about our loneliness, but to fuel our imagination and explore the corners of the earth in which we can still make a difference. And let us not forget to be grateful as we make all the farewells that we must make in due course – for the alternative to becoming old is not remaining young, but dying prematurely.

Decision-making conflicts

The older one gets, the more rigid one's habits become, and the more difficult it is to get rid of them if necessary. An established lifestyle usually proves to be quite persistent. This depends more on the lifestyle in question than on life experiences. Life experiences can be mildly formative or drastically life changing, but what comes from them and is decided in the light of them is astonishingly personal. People respond in completely different ways to almost identical experiences, and their responses may be anywhere on the scale between despair and laughter, or between submission and overcoming. One's lifestyle is formed from the sum of these responses.

Let's pick out one example: a man has to get up early in the morning to get to work. How does he respond to this situation? He can stay in bed until the last minute, stagger grumpily into the bathroom, gulp down a cup of coffee and rush out of the house with a deep sigh. Or he can begin the day in a completely different style. He can open his eyes and rejoice in seeing light and colours, grateful that he is not paralysed and can spring out of bed, grateful that he has a job and is not unemployed, and that the wonderful smell of fresh coffee will soon fill the kitchen. The situation is the same, but the response to it is very different, and accordingly the beginning of the day will feel very different.

Neuroscientists have long wondered whether the human brain preprograms our spontaneous reactions, or whether a person can really freely choose how to respond to life situations. There is now a widespread consensus that although the brain provides the burst of energy (degree of concentration and alertness) required to make decisions, it does not determine them. However little we can control the situation we are in, *we are free to choose how we respond to it!*

There is a small proviso. If we repeatedly make similar decisions in similar situations, a rigid automatism sets in. Our morning ritual, for example, is likely to take the same form for years on end. One no longer decides freely how to start the day, but surrenders oneself to this automatism. This has advantages and disadvantages. The advantage of fixed habits is to ease the burden of choice. It would simply be too complicated to always have to think about everything we do. It is like driving a car: with some practice, switching gears and operating the accelerator and brakes becomes automatic. The disadvantage is less activity of thought. In unusual situations, one cannot depend on habit and has to come up with novel responses, for which the required flexibility of thought may be lacking.

The best practice is therefore not to be driven blindly by habit, but to check from time to time whether habits are still appropriate or require changes. Inertia and the desire to do what is comfortable should not deprive us of the power to decide for ourselves! We need the competence to adapt to different stages of life, and that means discarding old decisions when necessary and replacing them with more appropriate ones. Even in cases of conflict (from which life does not spare us), we need the competence to give priority to the most meaningful option or lesser evil by means of decisively renouncing other options, so as not to be consumed by ambivalence.

To return to the morning routine: suppose the man wakes up with a sore throat and a fever. Should he call in sick with the consequence that he has to cancel important appointments, or should he drag himself into the office in his feverish state? One can only advise him to consider *everyone involved* as he makes this decision. To what extent will he endanger his health? How much will his customers suffer? How much extra work will fall on his colleagues? On the other hand, might he infect them? Those who have retained the elasticity of judgement required to make decisions without hesitation and in harmony with their conscience do not falter when they are conflicted. If the man decides to call in sick, in doing so he accepts the inconvenience to his customers and colleagues. If he decides to go to the office, he gives up the convenience of being able to look after himself. Every decision we make has a hook on which hangs a fragment of wistfulness. Every decision is a decision against something else that might also have been appealing. Thus, courage and wistfulness go hand in hand. Only by embracing this wistfulness are we able to act courageously, not allowing ourselves to be controlled by habits or paralyzed by a conflicted conscience.

Competitive pressure

In cases of confliction, I advised consideration of *everyone involved.* Why is it not enough to look after your own interests? Because this leads to even greater confliction. Egotistical behaviour widens the gap between us and other people and separates us from the community. And solitary confinement is the cruellest punishment of all. But what is our entrance ticket to the community? It is *doing as much good for others as for yourself.*

Frankl was a keen mountain climber, as he explained to the Olympic Games Committee in Munich in 1972. Properly understood, he said, competition pits us not against our competitors, but against ourselves. One attempts to optimize one's own skills – and that's all. The fear of lagging disgracefully behind others only dampens our enthusiasm. A mere stubborn determination to win puts a brake on success.

Frankl's warning is applicable to many areas of activity. If you focus on what others do better than you (or what they possess that you don't) you pull the ground from under your feet. It makes you look small, and envy and jealousy consume your soul. I used to ask my patients why they always compare themselves to tycoons and not to the millions of people who are much worse off than they are. That made them sit up and listen. *Actually, no comparisons with others should be permitted.* Every person is unique and has a different set of personal opportunities to make the most of his or her life. So parents should not compare their children with other children and they should resolutely oppose their children's desires to be given everything their classmates proudly show off to them. The fire of competitive pressure often ravages through schools, fuelling unpleasantnesses like bullying and scheming.

The best way to achieve your best is through flow experiences. As a result of the famous series of investigations by the American M. Csíkszentmihályi, we know that the strongest feelings of happiness and the most impressive achievements occur when people surrender in complete self-forgetfulness to a task that suits them and to which they are ardently committed. In these cases, the best "flows" out unintended, and what does happen is what cannot be directly targeted, namely rising above one's own limits. Paradoxically, in such moments of self-forgetfulness, human beings are at one with themselves more than ever. A part of the mystery of our ego is not to be

203

able to understand and grasp it by introspection – just as an astrono-mer on Earth can never view "Earth" through his telescope.

To prevent misunderstanding: a flow experience is not the same as working hard. Workaholism does not involve a healthy amount of *self-forgetfulness*, but it does forget *values in the outside world* that have a claim to consideration. An overworker ignores the body's warning signs. Family and friends are neglected, consideration for the environment is ignored, and in general, attention is withdrawn from everything but work. Such an individual becomes enmeshed in a fanatical zeal, which courts disaster like any fanaticism.

Let us therefore not impose work pressure on ourselves and oth-ers! Let us allow others their happiness, let us devote ourselves wholeheartedly to what we love, and let us beware of any kind of hyperintention, as Frankl called it. *What is ours will be successful, and what is not ours we can safely let go.*

Letting go

It is a psychologically absurd fact that the rich have greater problems with letting go than the poor. In the austere post-war period of my childhood, *twenty* children played with a ball possessed by *one* child. When the ball's owner grew up, the ball was given to a younger child. Toys were limited to a ball (and perhaps a teddy bear) and yet no one in our generation felt any lack. Today, in affluent countries, the talk is of sensory overload, and children can hardly escape from exciting gifts and diverse entertainment options. Between the bicker-ing of their parents, the horror stories on television, and the global apocalypses that filter into children's bedrooms, it is no surprise that fidgeting and provocation are increasingly common amongst chil-dren.

While sharing with one another is universal in conditions of pov-erty, greed is endemic in wealthy settings. Playing ball is a good symbol here: you have to *throw the ball back, or throw it to a play-mate* in order to free your hands to catch a ball again. If you hold on to the ball, you take yourself out of the game. Greedy people block themselves in a similar way. They squat in the midst of their abundance and the game of their own lives ebbs away. It is a sad warning sign that today we have houses full of junk, in which every drawer and attic corner is full of stuff that is no longer used and about which we have often completely forgotten. Piles of books are not read, CDs are not listened to, clothes are not worn, devices are ignored, but instead of getting rid of them, we shove them into basement rooms or even rent storage for them. This is the price one pays for wealth: a constant fear of losing one's riches and going under socially as well as materially. The poor, in contrast, have long since learned that their little canoe need not capsize even in shallow waters.

There is another disadvantage to excessive wealth. A lack of possessions fosters *creativity*. Children learn how to craft, paint, build fantastical objects from the humblest materials and occupy themselves quietly for hours. This ability is lost in a prefabricated "children's paradise". It has also been shown that adults have more and better ideas in simple surroundings, which is why artists like to retreat to remote places. Any overload reduces the capacity for thought; having too much gets in the way of simply being.

However, sooner or later life provides a correction and forces you to let go. None of our "possessions" are forever. Health deteriorates, relatives die, companions leave our side, professional responsibilities have to be passed on, economic circumstances deplete our bank account, and so on. In shock, one groans: "What is left?" Indeed, what is of lasting value?

We can circumnavigate the shock by practicing our ability to let go ahead of time. We can give away what we do not need. Let us strip our dwellings of everything unnecessary and content ourselves with a few rooms filled with light and air. With increasing population numbers and exploding city growth, it is unreasonable to hoard space. Let us watch our food and control our figure. Let us limit our leisure travel, and travel on foot as often as possible. Above all, however, let us let go inwardly of everything that has been granted to us over the years. *Even our loved ones,* if necessary. Let us throw back the ball, full of joy that we have been allowed to participate in the great game of life, aware that it was a sheer mercy to have loved and been loved.

What is left for us? *Only the truth about us,* and if it includes a spark of love, we have not lived in vain.

About the Authors

Prof. Elisabeth Lukas, PhD

Student of Viktor E. Frankl, clinical psychologist, psychotherapist, supervisor, speaker, honorary lecturer in the "original logotherapy according to Viktor E. Frankl", author of numerous specialist books which have been translated into 19 foreign languages. Many awards from universities and the city of Vienna for her services to the further development and dissemination of logotherapy.

Leopold-Gattringer-Str. 14/22, A 2345 Brunn am Gebirge

A current list of publications can be found at
www.elisabeth-lukas-archiv.de

Heidi Schönfeld, PhD

Student of Elisabeth Lukas, logotherapist, practicioner of psychotherapy and meaning-centred life counsellor active in her own practice. She is the founder and managing director of the Elisabeth-Lukas-Archive, to which an academy is affiliated. Speaker and lecturer in the subject of the "original logotherapy according to Viktor E. Frankl", supervisor, author, trainer in logotherapeutic counselling.

Nürnberger Str. 103a, D 96050 Bamberg

www.logotherapie-bamberg.de
www.elisabeth-lukas-archiv.de

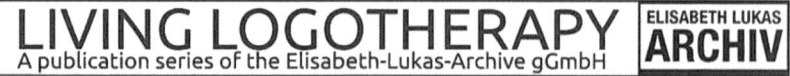

LIVING LOGOTHERAPY
A publication series of the Elisabeth-Lukas-Archive gGmbH

ELISABETH LUKAS
ARCHIV

MEANING-CENTRED PSYCHOTHERAPY
Viktor Frankl's Logotherapy in Theory and Practice
Elisabeth Lukas – Heidi Schönfeld

1. Edition: August 2019
ISBN: 9783000636004
e-Book-ISBN: 9783000642746

This book is a collaborative project. It combines discussions of the theory of logotherapy by Lukas with numerous case studies by Schönfeld. It gives readers a glimpse into the vitality and relevance of logotherapy.

LOGOTHERAPY
Principles and Methods
Elisabeth Lukas
1. Edition: September 2020
ISBN: 978-3-00-066678-0
e-Book-ISBN: 978-3-00-066679-7

The book provides a structured insight into Frankl's work. It explains the anthropological foundation of logotherapy and the healing concepts that are built on this foundation.